GO WITH YOUR GUT

THE INSIDER'S GUIDE TO
BANISHING THE BLOAT
WITH 75 DIGESTION-
FRIENDLY RECIPES

ROBYN YOUKILIS

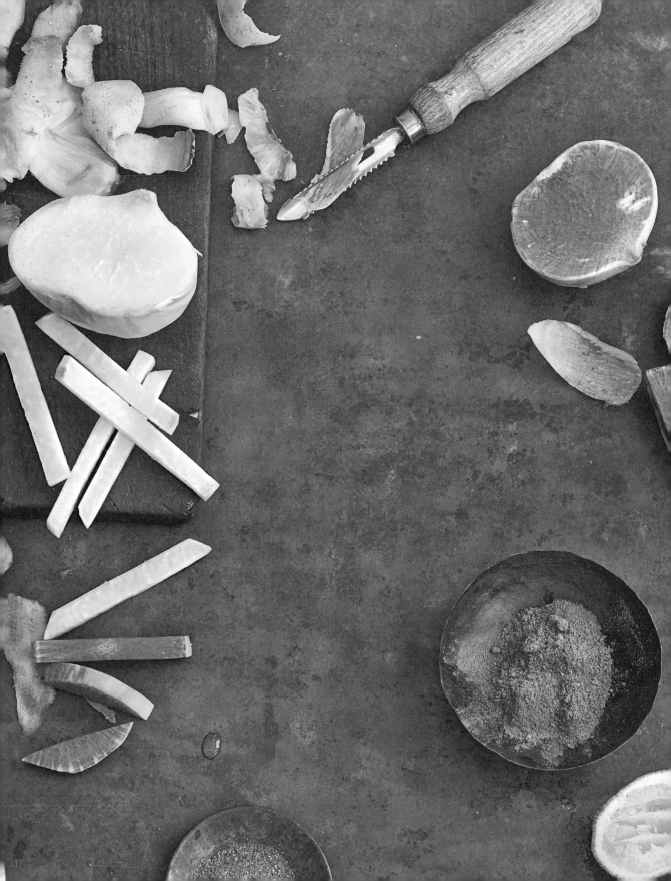

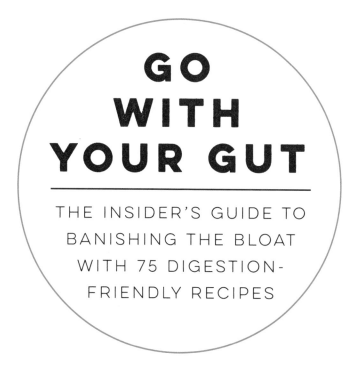

GO WITH YOUR GUT

THE INSIDER'S GUIDE TO BANISHING THE BLOAT WITH 75 DIGESTION-FRIENDLY RECIPES

ROBYN YOUKILIS

PHOTOGRAPHY BY

ELLEN SILVERMAN

KYLE BOOKS

This book is dedicated to you and your intuition,
that Sparkle in all of us.

★

May you be guided by your inner resource,
that purest place of you,
and watch your whole life expand.

First published in Great Britain in 2016 by
Kyle Books, an imprint of Kyle Cathie Ltd
192–198 Vauxhall Bridge Road
London SW1V 1DX
general.enquiries@kylebooks.com
www.kylebooks.co.uk

10 9 8 7 6 5 4 3 2 1

ISBN 978-0-85783-321-1

Project Editor: Jessica Goodman
Copy Editor: Ann Martin Rolke
Editorial Assistant: Claire Rogers
Angliciser: Anne McDowall
Designer: Nicky Collings
Photographer: Ellen Silverman
Food Stylist: Nora Singley
Prop Stylist: Alistair Turnbull
Production: Nic Jones, Gemma John and Lisa Pinnell

A Cataloguing in Publication record for this title is available
from the British Library.

Colour reproduction by ALTA London
Printed and bound in China by C&C Offset Printing Co., Ltd.

Important Note:
The information and advice contained in this book are intended
as a general guide and are not specific to individuals or
their particular circumstances. Neither the author nor the
publishers can be held responsible for claims arising from
the inappropriate use of any remedy or healing regime. Do
not attempt self-diagnosis or self-treatment for serious or
long-term conditions before consulting a medical professional
or qualified practitioner. Do not undertake any self-treatment
while taking other prescribed drugs or receiving therapy without
first seeking professional guidance. Always seek medical advice
if any symptoms persist.

CONTENTS

Foreword

Unlike most folks, I was brought up in a household that focused on homeopathic healing and digestive health. My family shopped only at health food shops, and we visited only acupuncturists, chiropractors and homeopaths when we were sick. I rarely took antibiotics and I was taught to meditate and practise mindfulness from a very young age.

You'd think that with such a great upbringing in holistic healing that I'd have it all together by the time I was an adult. Well, that wasn't the case. By the time I was in my mid-twenties I was burnt out, detoxing from drugs and alcohol, confused about what to eat and feeling sick all the time. I was in desperate need of inspiration and guidance.

Then, right when I needed her most, I was reconnected with my old college friend Robyn Youkilis. We reunited in Los Angeles at a small talk I was giving. At the time, I was beginning my career as a speaker and an author, and Robyn came out to support me. She was also involved in the world of personal growth: she had just graduated from the Institute for Integrative Nutrition and launched an awesome career as a health coach and wellness maven. That night in L.A., we began a journey that in time turned into a treasured friendship. We connected deeply through our shared love for healing, spirituality and health. We became each other's spiritual running buddies and confidants. But little did I know that Robyn would one day be my gut guru.

Over time, she began to gently guide me towards greater physical health. Whenever I'd join her for a meal, she would kindly offer tips on how I could adjust my eating. Without any judgment, Robyn would lovingly help me witness my food behaviour and how it was not serving me. She'd watch me shovel food down my throat so that I could get to the next meeting or reply to an email. She'd say, 'G! Your stomach doesn't have teeth'. Robyn would tell me what to order at a restaurant to ensure that I was combining foods in the right way. And she'd spend countless hours walking me through the grocery store to make sure I went home with all the right ingredients to support my precious gut. Best of all, Robyn became my personal recipe book. Whenever I wanted to whip up a creative, delicious and healthy dinner, she would text me the ingredients while I was walking to the grocery store. Having Robyn on my speed dial has saved my meals and my digestive system!

I'm so happy that this book is in your hands because now you, too, can know the divine blessing of having your very own gut guru. In this book, Robyn tackles one of the most important health issues of our time – gut health. I can personally testify to this. Throughout my life I suffered from acne, foggy brain, mild depression, lethargy and a poor immune system – until I started healing the flora in my gut. Committing to cleansing my gut and then rebuilding the natural flora cleared up my skin completely, reenergised me and boosted my immune system to the point where I never get sick. I swear by the fact that a healthy gut creates a healthy life.

You picked up this book because there is a subtle voice within you beckoning you to clean up your act. You have a powerful opportunity to turn your health around. This is not just another diet book – this is a pathway to true healing. If you're ready to go big and own your power, then GO WITH YOUR GUT!

My soul sister Robyn will offer you everything you need on your divine journey towards healing. Plus, there is no one in the world who can be quite so cute, brilliant and respectable while saying the word 'poop'!

Enjoy this healing journey and expect miracles!

Gabrielle Bernstein
New York Times **bestseller author of** *Miracles Now*

INTRODUCTION

I would bet you a green juice that you don't know all the bodily functions that are affected by your digestive system. Most of us have no idea how much the health of our bellies impacts our lives and bodies, and until I went to the Institute for Integrative Nutrition (IIN) – where I became a holistic nutritional coach and a member of AADP (the American Association of Drugless Practitioners) – I honestly didn't think about it either.

I am fully convinced that there is a reason why our bellies are located in the centre, or core, of our bodies. The health of your digestive system influences everything – energy, mental focus, mood and appearance (hair, skin, nails, weight). The better your body is able to process and use the nutrients from your food, the better you feel. Not to mention that your digestion plays a big part in how often you get sick and how often your body can take out the rubbish. Taking it a step further, I believe there is a connection between a powerfully functioning gut and a powerfully functioning 'gut instinct'. When the belly is at its healthiest, we can hear those gut messages loud and clear. How we digest our food is how we digest our lives. And my ladies, when our insides and outsides are in sync, it's like we are covered in sparkle dust – the best of who we are gets turned up ten notches.

Throughout the past 6 years in my client practice with Your Healthiest You, I've helped thousands of people around the world learn to live free of the craziness of dieting and connect to what I call their 'sparkle'. I've become totally absorbed in practising, through trial and error, what I preach and constantly taking in every morsel from the teachers and sages of my industry.

My clients rely on me to teach them the way through the emotional and physical challenges they face every day. But the dirty truth is, it wasn't long ago that I was really miserable in my own skin. I was constantly trying to find the trick that would fix me. I swore off all breads and carbs forever one month. I attempted to skip out on my friends' invitations to dinner the next. I tried to live solely on green drinks and smoothies and, even though I totally knew better, I took 'holistic' supplements that promised to help me lose weight.

When I was working in Los Angeles as an actress, I eventually went to Weight Watchers and I did lose weight. I was fed up with my body and how I couldn't seem to keep myself from raiding the kitchen cabinets at night. I found myself obsessing about dieting and my body even more than I had before. And since maths is not my forté, I certainly didn't want to have to count points for the rest of my life. How could I limit myself to eating boring salads when there is so much delicious food out there to be eaten? Through and through, I am a foodie at heart, and I knew enough to see that if the diet felt so at odds with who I was in my gut, I was never going to stick to it.

No matter what crazy diet I tried, deep down I felt that my outside was not a reflection of who I knew myself to be on the inside. What I discovered is that when I tried to fix my outside, I was exhausted by the constant chatter going on in my brain: 'Is it okay to eat that? What if I just have a little? Oh, this cheese/wine/dessert is staring at me, I'll just have one more bite. God, you suck! Well, we'll start again tomorrow!' I was carrying around excess pounds of emotional and physical baggage. I didn't even know where to begin.

I'd panic when the jeans that were supposed to fit were too tight and I had to go up yet another size. I had categories of jeans for the heavier me and for the slimmer me instead of one wardrobe for one girl. I was always stressing about food, exercise and whether my clothes were properly positioned to hide the little belly that was uncomfortably hanging over the top of my trousers. My day was a constant 'adjust my blouse to cover my belly' fixation.

Does this sound familiar? It's soooo exhausting, right?

These obsessions with weight, diet, exercise and even health don't have to be a part of everyday life. Anyone can change their relationship with food and their body. We need to slow down, start from the beginning and actually look at what's going on here. We need to focus on what our symptoms are telling us. We all have this innate wisdom inside of us. And through the guidance in this book, the communication between you and your gut will become clear.

There is no greater motivator for a girl than to just be freaking thin already. Done with it. Thin was an answer to all happiness, finding the man I could be worthy of, if only I lost those 10 to 15 pounds that make me look like Bridget Jones instead of Renee Zellweger.

So those 15 bloody pounds (ok, fine, 20) didn't go anywhere. I could not seem to make the connection for myself between knowing and being. I could not figure out the connection with my behaviour; the flow from brain to body to belly, from 'I should' to 'this is what I do'.

And then, there it was in the same way that all great things have come to me in my life. Every clear decision I've ever made has come from a place in my gut, from that intuitive place of knowing we all describe, for no reason we can explain, as coming from the depth of our tummies. When something is off, that place becomes a hard, tight pit. When something is right, it dances and sparkles; it is that inarguable YES. It happened to me the moment I looked up and saw my husband Scott for the first time. It happened when I held the brochure to IIN, the school where I ended up studying nutrition, in my hand. I proceeded to figure out exactly how to pay the tuition and move from Los Angeles back to New York within a week. Every clear, right and best next step in my life has come from that place of knowing. I knew this as a child, too. And if you have kids they do too. But over time, I clouded it with fear, stress, anxiety and bad food behaviours – from packaged, processed foods and sugar to all the sugar-free, low-calorie or fat-free 'diet' foods I was consuming daily – until my abilities became a fogged-up mess. In my search for what was missing for me and those I was trying to help, from answering the question of 'What am I not getting here?' to 'What do I need?', I discovered what made the most sense to me and it turns out to be as basic as it gets. It's all about the link I make between our literal guts and our gut. Taking it one step further, our intuition.

All that I have achieved in my adult life is a result of cleaning up my food and cleaning up my gut, therefore being able to live my life from that place of intuition – because everything is flowing, moving and clear. (And yes, we are pooping well, too.) We feel good about who we are being.

I knew in my gut where every aspect of our well-being generates from and returns to – our bellies. There's a whole lot of science out there on this and you could read it yourself, but it's my mission to break it down for you. This is all intended for someone who takes their life seriously and wants to know their shit (literally). We are so cut off from our bodies and our bellies, but really it can be so straightforward, direct and simple. You already have everything you need to do this and do it every day. This is your girlfriend's no-nonsense, go-to guide to taking care of the part of you that takes care of the rest of you.

My *Go With Your Gut* teachings have helped my clients begin to resolve their stubborn food issues in a matter of weeks – without having to go on a 'diet'. Diets wreak havoc on your digestive system. My programme puts the focus on maximising good digestive habits, which not only has the potential to make you feel spectacular, but also helps to heal the body from the inside out.

Best of all, I am not asking you to be 'perfect' in order to feel and look better. Once you get your digestion back on track through establishing amazing digestive habits, you will be able to enjoy food pleasures without a recurrence of symptoms or any of the mental drama that comes with what we traditionally refer to as a 'diet'. As one of my clients posted on our group Facebook support page, 'The best part was not thinking, "I shouldn't have this." It was just a decision I made … there was no further inner discussion about it!'

Here's the secret to the success of *Go With Your Gut*; once you decide to live your life more healthily, your brain is free of all that 'should I/shouldn't I?' chatter. This translates into being able to truly commit to, show up for and be passionate about life. One of my clients recently wrote to me about how her life had been completely transformed, saying, 'I know which foods feel best for me and which ones I want to have less of. I'm looking at this program as a guide for a daily routine that makes me feel like a rockstar every day, while still having room for real life.' Personally, after living *Go With Your Gut* for a while now, I feel the same way. Hundreds of my clients have seen the same transformation in their lives – just by improving their digestive health.

One of the best benefits of the *Go With Your Gut* lifestyle is the ability to enjoy the foods you love but still wake up feeling energised and looking great the next day. When you have a routine to follow and aren't worried about 'slipping up', activities like travelling and eating out become completely drama-free.

In each chapter, I give a specific 'Practice' you can follow in order to help you get the most out of this experience. (I'll cover cravings, bloating and energy, just to name a few.) The simple strategies I provide will help you resolve those daily issues and symptoms, from constipation to acid reflux.

Everything I advise in this book is easy, affordable and doesn't require you to skip your favourite 4-hour brunch gabfest on Sundays. Or forgo your beloved local restaurant. Or never eat a slice of delicious bread again.

So, let's get real here. You picked up this book because you want to poop more, be less bloated – which is probably code for 'I am fat' (at least you think so) – and be the ultimate you (whether that means 'thin' or something else). We will seemingly do anything to get thin – cigarettes, diet sodas, packets upon packets of artificial sweetener. We have even started trying to outsmart our bodies with pseudo-healthy habits like rigid juice cleanses or the latest supplement fad or worse.

Every pill you put in your mouth, from antibiotics to a herbal supplement, has a direct effect on your digestive system. But knowing what not to do just isn't enough. As I show you what to focus on instead – what I often refer to as 'upgrading' from a harmful habit to one that both helps and works – you will find that you no longer need to reach for those things that are hurting your belly, mind and soul.

My philosophy is about the whole body, the whole person from top to toe, and that includes the emotional you. It's about practising gentleness and supporting your strengths. It also is NOT about perfection. Sometimes you're on top of it; sometimes not so much. It's all okay. And all a part of being human.

We all rebel against what we know is best for us. Anyone familiar with me on social media knows that I have my moments when I just say 'eff-it' to my normal non-negotiables. The key is to let loose without losing yourself completely. It is not about never indulging. For example, while I may stay up an hour or two later than usual, I don't keep myself awake until 2am. And while I may have an extra glass of wine, I'm sure to not make it two extra. I still eat chocolate and yummy desserts. But it's chocolate without added crappy sugars, and I think it tastes better (and feels better). Most importantly, though, I don't sacrifice my standards. Even when I'm indulging a bit more than usual, I don't slip back into eating crap. Because that never makes me feel good.

When you're cooking my recipes throughout the week, you're covered. When you are slowly but surely creating daily habits out of the easy lifestyle changes I lay out for you, finding your body's natural weight is going to become a by-product. You will be thin from within.

You will also be well. You will be able to think clearly without your brain and body being bogged down by using its forces to process what it can't. You will have higher energy, be tooting and burping less, your skin will glow, your eyes will sparkle ... you will sparkle – your whole, entire being.

Remember, what we're aiming for here is a 'most-of-the-time' improvement. Each small step will build on the next one. The better you start to feel, the more you will find yourself relying on these new habits and releasing the old. Is your diet and emotional well-being better most of the time? Then that, my dear, is success.

We are going to start with the basics of belly knowledge: the who, what and where. Then we will get to your new non-negotiables: chewing, water, breathing. These are so hugely graspable and have such an enormous impact. You are going to start feeling incredible. I can't wait.

AN INTRODUCTION TO THE RECIPES

Whenever I cook, I first ask myself, '*what do I want?*'

This is the start of the conversation I have with my belly and my body. Do I want animal protein today? Do I feel like making a whole dish? Or do I just want to throw something together quickly? Do I want to eat out of a bowl? Something light and crunchy? Or heavy and warm? Spicy? Salty? Sweet? And the questions go on and on…

This might sound like a lot of extra time or even crazy.

But actually, it's kind of crazy that we don't have this conversation with ourselves. We cook what we know, order whatever sounds good in that moment or hand over the choosing to someone else.

None of this is bad or wrong, it's just that asking yourself what YOU really want and need is the start to fixing YOUR digestion and connecting to your total 'you-ness': that intuitive place inside that knows exactly what your body (and life) is asking for. After a while, this will become automatic (and has probably already happened many times, like when you choose soup on a cold, winter day).

Once you start the conversation, listen for the answer – and then do (or make) what your body is asking for.

These recipes were created with exactly that kind of thinking in mind. What do you need? What sounds amazing to you? Always keep fresh, lively produce around and stock your pantry with the recipe staples so you'll be able to make anything from this book at any time.

The recipes are located at the end of each chapter, so as you expand your knowledge, you'll also expand your cooking repertoire. They fit with the themes of the chapters, but also stand entirely on their own.

I encourage you to read through all of them before cooking anything. This way you'll have a strong sense of what's in here – and you'll be much more likely to use it. I've designed *Go With Your Gut* to be beautiful and sit elegantly on your coffee table or nightstand, but my real goal is for you to get it as dirty as possible in your kitchen. I give you full permission to write all over the pages, dog ear the recipes you can't wait to make or draw a star near or highlight any points or helpful tips you want to be able to come back to easily. Let it be the space to chronicle your personal journey to a happier belly and body.

This book is your playground.

Love it up and you'll be able to live it up.

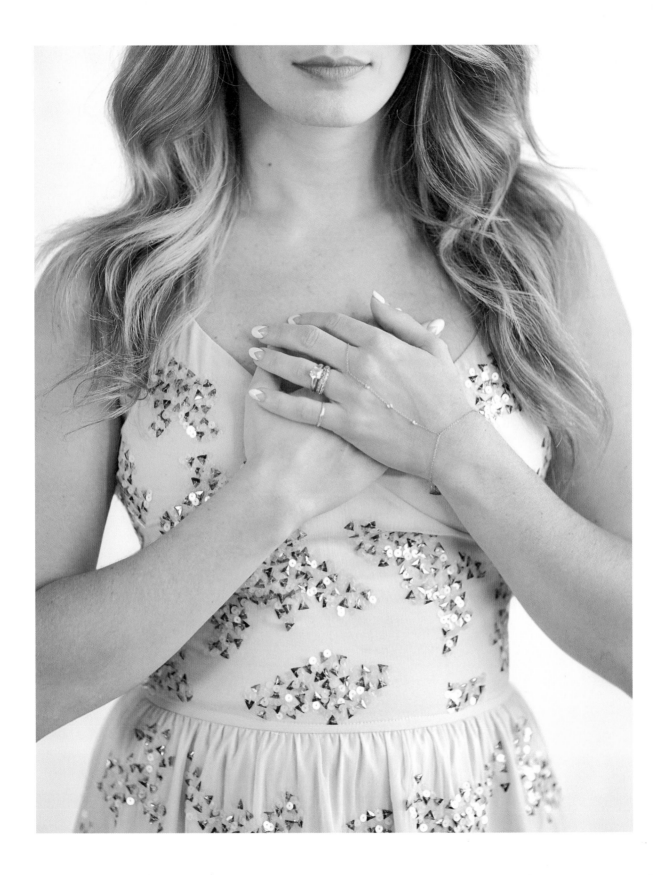

CHAPTER 1

BREATHE

A thriving digestive system has the power to give us all the good things we want: dewy, blemish-free skin, strong hair and nails, bouncy energy, restful sleep, relief from ailments and, yes, a trim little waistline. If the lives of my clients are anything to go by, most of us are experiencing our day-to-day with unhappy bellies and some form of digestive dysfunction.

Bad digestion is about skipping lunch for a work call. It's about taking that call with a pit in your stomach while thinking, 'I have to get that urgent email out!' It's about following that missed meal hours later by overdoing the guacamole and tortilla chips before dinner is served at the restaurant, because you're starving. It's realising you ate an entire container of hummus while watching an episode of *Scandal* or *Real Housewives* without even noticing. (Quick tip: think dip instead of dunk!). It's being too tired to go to the gym or yoga. It's about your 3pm latte that you need to stay awake after lunch. It's going to Happy Hour with your girlfriends in order to drink to forget instead of to connect and laugh. It's always eating on the go. It's feeling like you are constantly running on fumes. It's that 'ugh' feeling on a weekday morning and your usual hangover or couch collapse on Sunday.

Issues with your body can be the result of constantly ruminating on what you ate and where it's going to show up as fat tomorrow. A lack of nutrients and the inability to slow down and truly rest can cause you to wake up and wonder if you slept at all. Your gut can make you feel like your body is fighting against you, day in and day out.

The helpless feeling of not knowing what causes our symptoms leads to us trying a million different things to get fast results, such as acid reflux medicines and even laxatives. We try probiotics, but the wrong ones. We take supplements that we lack the digestive function to absorb. We try a new diet that we read about online, even though we know that we can't maintain it when it leaves us feeling deprived. We start a juice cleanse every few weeks, spend all our money on elite weightloss services and then give up within the first 24 hours. With what a friend of mine jokingly called 'the Upper East Side solution' in New York City, we mechanically eliminate gluten, dairy and sugar because it worked for our friends, without thinking about our own bodies. We go to our doctor and they don't know what's up. Or worse yet, they prescribe us meds that we're not really sure we want or need. We blame it on our genes. We blame it on our food sensitivities. We wonder why we feel so crappy when we're trying so hard to do all the right things.

As you learn to take care of your whole body, through the foundation of understanding how to care for your remarkable belly, you will see that what I say is true – everything becomes better when we fix the one thing that impacts everything: our digestion.

So where have we been going wrong?

THE LINK BETWEEN STATE OF MIND AND STATE OF BELLY

So many of us walk around in a state of unfriendly belly. And there are so many different ways the problem can start. Maybe it's with one negative, such as a sour stomach every time we were afraid as a child or an idea that 'I have always had sinus issues; that's just who I am'. We become so accustomed to the effects of our daily dysfunction that we start to ignore them. It gets to the point when we don't even notice that first symptom or we pass it off because it's so familiar. Well, there are healthy ways to treat these routine problems before they become big ones. And guess what? Those routine problems have everything to do with your digestion.

I want to be able to tell you that I never experienced a dysfunctional relationship with my belly. I wish I could tell you that I sat down to write this book from a place of perfection, that I grew up in a house where I was raised from infancy to make the right choices and just kept getting wiser from there. That I was always one of those girls who was ready to throw her bikini in a bag and run to the beach with the boys without wishing I'd had a month of extreme behaviour, gym time and crash dieting beforehand. Sorry, but no way.

By emotionally twisting ourselves into knots, we are doing our waistlines and our well-being no favours. I want you to start thinking about your state of mind as a key part of your digestion. Whether it's going through your entire day feeling anxious about your weight or any of the other million reasons we come up with to feel stressed and unsettled, we begin at square one on a shaky foundation.

Think about what you have been stressing out about today. I bet the list comes up in your mind pretty fast. How does that make you feel in your stomach? Now think about something that brings you peace, joy and ease. What did your belly do then? Did it release and relax? Did your breath naturally start to feel more full? The power of our mind and its connection to our belly is immense.

How many times has an anxious day or fight with your mum/friend/co-worker led you to binge on the entire contents of your fridge the moment you were alone? The habits that mess with our digestion show up in so many different ways.

So, what are you ignoring?

These symptoms are huge signs from the universe that something is up with your body and that you desperately need a change. The only – and I mean only – way to begin to change is to start small. I mean teeny, tiny, baby steps small.

Here is where better digestion begins: from the simplest possible place. You don't need any ingredients or kitchen gadgets to create it; it's a thought. Instead of telling yourself you are behind, too late, inadequate, I want you to tell yourself that you are exactly as you are supposed to be. The knowledge you are going to take on throughout this book will support and deepen that feeling.

It is scientifically accepted that when we experience stress or emotional disturbance, it affects our cortisol levels, which in turn affects our blood sugar levels and the brain's ability to communicate smoothly with the digestive system. Can you imagine what you do to your stomach when you are in a constant state of peaks and valleys?

Consequently, science is all over the link between cortisol and weight gain. Cortisol has been dubbed the 'stress hormone' and, as with most overblown media coverage aimed to make you scared of your body, you're supposed to freak out now. Don't! Here is what it does: your adrenal glands secrete it, it metabolises glucose, regulates your blood pressure, releases insulin for blood sugar maintenance, supports your immune function and regulates your inflammatory response.

There is nothing wrong with your body producing cortisol as a response to a moment of stress. That's what it's supposed to do. The problem is when you spend all day in a state of frenzy and the stress just doesn't stop – you are then in a state of imbalance. Your body can't tell the difference between the stress of leaving your beloved make-up case on the subway and the stress of encountering a mama bear and her cubs during a run near a farm (both of which happened to me in the same two weeks, by the way). All your body knows is there is stress, danger, a threat. Now your thoughts become scattered and you can't think straight; your thyroid is all jacked up; you can be hyperglycemic or just plain up and down with your blood sugar; and your bone density isn't

great. You also can get high blood pressure, your immunity is weaker and, yes, your fat cell levels can increase and muscle tissue can be affected.

Bottom line: I want you to train yourself how to return from a state of imbalance to balance. In the beginning, you may have to do the practices I teach you 20 times a day. But over time, it will become easier and easier. You don't want your cortisol level to spike unless they are supposed to. You don't want your body to be in a state of prolonged red-alert. We are not hunter-gatherers anymore and our sense of danger often comes from emotional triggers rather than mortal danger, yet the body only recognises what you tell it: danger is danger.

So, our emotions are a big part of our belly life. We have to consider this as part of the whole belly megillah. With that in mind, I have some homework for you.

THE SIMPLE POWER OF BREATHING

The very first thing you can start to do during your day to aid your belly is begin to learn how to talk to yourself more effectively and how to focus on your breathing.

Anyone who has taken a yoga class knows that breath is indeed impactful to our entire bodies. By just fully inhaling, with your mind focused on your breath rather than the million other cares and worries of your day, you can slow down your heart rate. But it's not automatic. When you are under stress, your breath becomes shorter, shallower, less oxygenating. Limited or dysfunctional breathing alone can cause you to hyperventilate.

Have you ever been in a yoga class and thought, 'Am I actually doing anything? Am I burning enough fat? I should have done cardio instead –

this is so slow!' And then the next day you're all glowy and shiny and your tummy seems flatter and your muscles feel stretched in the best places. In focusing on your breathing, you can cause yourself to sweat. If you can make water come out of your body and appear suddenly on the tip of your nose, can you imagine what learning to be more aware of your breathing throughout your day can do to your digestion? I mean, it's major! And this is before you even get close to thinking about or dealing with food. By changing your breathing throughout your day you make a huge impact on your digestive system.

A question that I frequently ask my clients is whether they check in with themselves throughout the day. What I mean by this is whether we all talk to ourselves. How you do it, though, is a big deal. Do you ask yourself questions about what you think, what you want, how you feel? Do you pause and listen in order to address the answers that come to you? What if you allowed yourself a full two weeks, before you go anywhere near the fork factor, to start becoming aware of your breath more often? For example, imagine your boss just embarrassed you at a meeting simply to make them look good. Do you stop and say, 'I'm so furious right now. My face feels hot and my ears are red. I need to take three deep breaths. I need to slow down. Just breathe, girl. In and out'. Or do you hold on tight to that shortened breath state, steamrolling through the rest of the day from that place, making one less-than-healthy choice after the next?

This is a perfect example of when those 'fight or flight' hormones kick in. You have the ability to influence how this plays out. You can positively or negatively affect how your body reacts to the food you give it an hour or so after the mentally upsetting incident. What you wind up craving, and how powerful those cravings

can feel, can be changed by you becoming more aware of your breath and by asking questions that are focused not on criticism but on the practical and basic. How do I feel? If your answer is 'I'm so insanely stressed', or even if it's 'I'm mildly tense about whether I should book my holiday plane tickets before I leave work today', then right then, you can do this exercise:

★ Place your hand on your heart.

★ Breathe in and out. Full, deep inhalation. Expand the belly, breathing into your lower back and sides. Then make a full, long exhalation, with a complete emptying of the lungs.

★ Become aware of the expression on your face. Are your lips tight and severe? What about that space between your eyebrows? Use your mind. Imagine your face softening.

★ What is happening in your shoulders? In your neck? Take it down your body. Take stock of what is happening down to your toes.

★ As you get in touch with each part of your body, from your scalp to your feet, ask if you can release a little bit more.

★ Relaxing can be whatever you like – make it up based on what feels right to you. But use it. Go to it.

If you think you have a high-octane job and urgent responsibilities and can't realistically take time out when things get intense, just consider that this is all about helping you be more effective and more powerful with your time. This will help you move through your busy day in a better way! There is always time to relax a little and put yourself in a slightly better mood. Breathing, smiling, checking in: these habits make us feel better. Plus, with practice,

I promise this can take you just 2 minutes. At a yoga vacation my husband Scott and I attended, Domenic, one of my favourite teachers, used the yogic expression, 'If you're not breathing, you're just posing'. In other words, if you're not breathing, you're not actually practising yoga.

Yoga aside, breathing deeply and fully in as many moments as possible is the kind of small shift that begins with awareness and can end up with profoundly significant reverberations to your health and longevity. Once you are at the point of catching yourself in a moment holding your breath because you are scared or upset and you become conscious of it and make a change, you are doing it.

And yes, this all matters when it comes to food. Same day, same office and it's birthday cupcake time. Check in! 'Hello, Robyn, I'm here. How are you? Stop. Breathe. Relax. Here is my breath; here is my stomach.' Place one hand on your heart, the other on your belly. You might want to step into an empty conference room in case someone sees you and thinks you're nuts, but whatever. Ask yourself, 'Am I hungry right now? What was I going to eat for lunch? Will I want my lunch if I eat this cupcake right now?'

What is going on in your head right now as you reach for this cake? Maybe you were part of a big family with a lot of siblings all crowded around the same dinner table. Maybe you used to worry that if everyone reached for the plate of food at once there would be none left for you. Maybe the energy was frenetic and excited as you ate. That was then; this is now. Is your heart rate elevated? Are you feeling an competitive animal instinct in order to ensure that you get one? Do you even WANT the bloody cupcake?

This will not lead to over-thinking and becoming overly conscious while you interact with your food. You are already obsessed with what you eat. We all are. I WANT to raise your level of consciousness as you eat. It's not a negative thing to be mindful. It's just a matter of how. Or, as one of my clients once said so brilliantly, 'It's a matter of being conscious, not crazy!' I don't want you to scoff or be distracted and forget that you ate at all. I want you to see, smell, taste and, yes, think about what you're eating. I promise it won't make you neurotic.

The 123 Food Freedom Tool is a practice I created that I come back to constantly because I know if I just tell myself, 'Be more mindful when eating!' it doesn't always work. I need a specific technique, a system that I can follow without having to think about it so much.

Think for a moment about the actual experience of eating. Sometimes it's relaxed and for enjoyment and nourishment, but most of the time it's hurried and we don't even completely know we're eating. And then we're finished and we wonder, 'Where did my food go? And why do I want MORE?' And that's when you end up back in the fridge or continuing to work your way through an entire container of kale chips.

★

123 FOOD FREEDOM TOOL

STEP ONE
LOOK AT YOUR PLATE

STEP TWO
BREATHE

STEP THREE
CHEW

First up, go and grab a piece of food. It only needs to be a couple of bites. Bring it back to your seating area.

Now look at your food. I can totally feel you rolling your eyes, but think about it for a moment. When was the last time you allowed your eyes to take in the experience of eating? Eating is a complete sensory experience and if we don't include one of our most vital senses, our sight, we are out of touch with the idea that we have eaten. You only have to do it for a second, and even if it's an on-the-go bar or apple I want you to look at it.

If you forget to use this tool at the start of your meal, you can stop eating at any time and do it! When I sometimes forget, I will put the food or my fork down and start over with Step One.

Now breeeathe. Taking a breath brings you back to the present and allows you to feel like you're in your body again (which is necessary because you're about to use your body to eat!). This works no matter where you're eating: the subway, car, desk – anywhere. Take a pause and take a good breath, and I mean a real breath, not a short silly one. Do you feel calmer? How foreign does that feel? As it turns out, deep breathing is not only relaxing, it's been scientifically proven by studies at the Cleveland Clinic's Center for Integrative Medicine to affect the heart, the brain, digestion and the immune system.

When we hold our breath, which we do constantly without awareness, the physical response is to cut off the air supply between our lungs or lower half of our bodies and our head. When we're cut off from our bodies, we're cut off from the experience of eating.

Another important point here: Even if you're eating something that you would rather not, whatever that is for you (bagels, ice cream, etc.), I still want you to look at it and practise the 123 Food Freedom Tool.

Chew! Chewing is so important that I've devoted the entire next chapter to this subject. For this practice, chew each mouthful completely before swallowing. We are going to dig way into exactly how to chew, what it does for your belly and your body in Chapter 2. See you there!

★

I created the 123 Food Freedom Tool for when life is a bit hectic and you're distracted during your meal. Whether it's kids, the phone or emails, this tool allows you to check in and slow down so you can savour.

BREATHE RECIPES

Let's kick off your plan by starting with the most important meal of the day – breakfast! I love how breakfast is the first way I can say, 'Robyn, I am going to take care of you today. I'm going to think about what you need and how I can fuel you.' Breakfast is an opportunity to get your belly going in the right direction and each good choice leads to the next. Your belly loves breakfast too! A warm, nourishing breakfast gets your brain zinging and your cells flowing.

As far as flavours go, I love them all – the sweet, the savoury, the bitter, the tart – and I've found a way to give you the rich and hearty tastes we long for.

Superhuman Breakfast
Superhuman Breakfast Frittata
Overnight Oats
Amaranth Porridge
Apple Chia Cereal
Eggs and Oats
Sweet Cinnamon Scramble
Chia Cakes
Sweet Cinnamon Sauce
Nut Butter Sauce

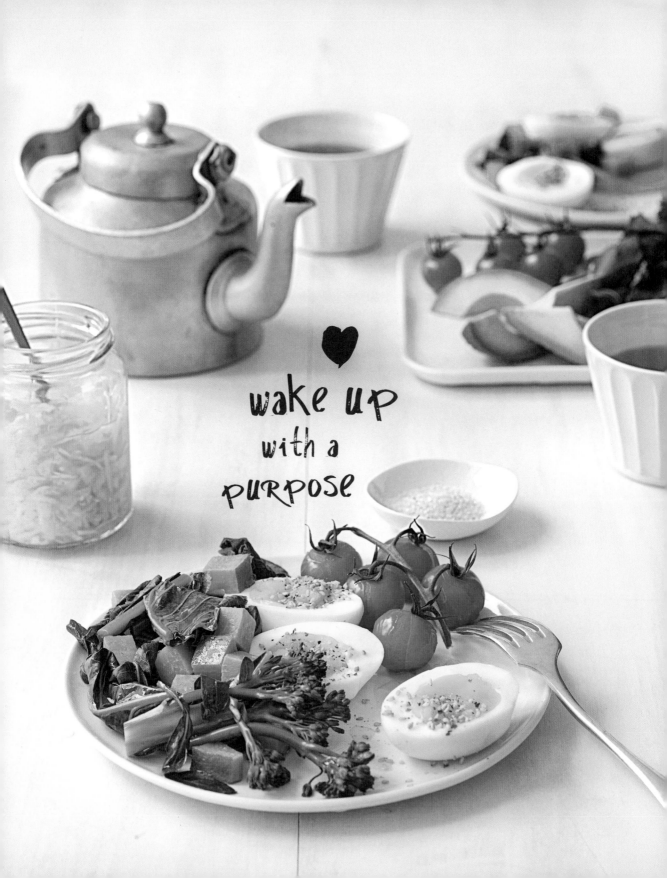

wake up
with a
purpose

SUPERHUMAN BREAKFAST

Ahh the 'superhuman breakfast'. The cornerstone of the Go With Your Gut *plan, this meal was THE game changer for me. It stimulated so many other amazing changes in my body. I used to make smoothies or green juices because I thought I needed something 'light' in the morning. I thought my 'iffy' stomach couldn't properly digest whole foods in their original form, meaning I chose blended raw over steamed kale. I was wrong. Rather than waking my gut with cold liquid, it needed a warm and grounding meal to get going; something that would really satisfy me, and not just for a couple of hours.*

This meal was created and coined by one of my teachers and dear friends, Laura Hames Franklin, founder of the School of Universal Health Principles and School for Superhumans (hence the breakfast name!).

I look forward to eating this breakfast (almost) every day. And with all the variations, it never gets old. You can mix it up with different kinds of sweet potatoes, herbs, kraut and, best of all, who you eat it with. My favourite way to enjoy it is on the weekends when my hubby and I can slow down and enjoy the food and being together.

FOR EACH SERVING

100–200g starchy veg: sweet potato, squash

2 eggs: boiled, poached, steamed, scrambled or fried – and eat the yolks too! Note: if you don't eat eggs you can swap them with a piece of tempeh (a fermented soybean cake) or a small piece of fish, but really any whole protein source will work (soaked and cooked beans, chicken, etc.)

Unlimited greens: kale, collards (my favourite!), spinach and broccoli
Optional additional veggies: mushrooms, tomatoes and zucchini, or anything that's fresh, abundant and in-season.

Up to **100g** fermented veggies (raw and unpasteurised): sauerkraut, kimchi, or any fermented vegetables

How to create and bring this beautiful meal together:

1 Gather all your ingredients, a cutting board and a knife. Wash anything that needs to be washed.

2 Next fill a medium to large saucepan with 5cm of water, fit the pan with a steamer basket and set over high heat on the hob, covered with a lid. If you are poaching or boiling your eggs, you'll want to fill an additional pan of water and set it on the hob to boil.

3 While your water begins to boil, chop about 100g worth of your starchy veggie (up to 200g if you find you are hungry sooner than three hours after consuming this meal) into a small dice. (The smaller the chop the quicker it will cook!) Once your water is boiling (steam is coming out of the pan), add your starchy veggies to the steamer basket. If you are boiling your eggs, gently add them to the water and set your timer for 7 minutes for a soft, runny yolk or 8–9 minutes for a soft to firmer, less runny yolk.

SUPERHUMAN BREAKFAST CONTINUED

Additional add-ons: drizzle of olive, hemp, or pumpkin seed oil; avocado; sprinkle of gomasio (sesame salt) or sesame seeds; fresh herbs such as oregano, thyme or rosemary; Himalayan pink sea salt; black pepper; cayenne pepper

NOTE

Ideally your breakfast will contain each of the main four components of this meal: eggs, greens, starchy veggie and fermented veggies or sauerkraut.

The rest is up to you and your imagination!

The Superhuman Breakfast may seem like a lot to do at first within an hour of waking up - especially if you're used to pouring some flakes in a bowl and adding milk or skipping breakfast entirely. I suggest starting on a weekend day when you may have more time and feel more relaxed in the kitchen. After you make it a few times it will become like a dance you look forward to.

4 Next, tear and prep your greens or chop any additional veggies you'll be using and add them to the steamer pot on top of your starchy veggies.

5 If you are scrambling, poaching or frying your eggs you'll want to begin that part now.

6 Test your veggies – you should easily be able to poke a fork through everything in the steamer. Once cooked, remove veggies with tongs and place on your serving plate(s).

7 Remove eggs from the saucepan or frying pan, depending on cooking method, and peel or place on plate with veggies.

8 Add a few forkfuls of fermented veggies to the plate and garnish with fresh herbs. If using your favourite healthy fat (a drizzle of oil, ¼ – ½ an avocado) – you'll want to experiment with how much or how little fat you use depending on hunger levels and how you feel after your breakfast. Some days I need a little more, some days a little less. Check in with how you're feeling and what your intuition is saying to you. Season generously with salt, pepper and any additional spices.

9 Serve immediately and eat!

For an on-the-go option you can place your Superhuman Breakfast items in a reusable glass container.

Want to see a video of me prepping this meal? Head to www.robynyoukilis.com/gutbookbonuses for an ingredient tutorial and a few fun variations on this incredible breakfast!

SUPERHUMAN BREAKFAST FRITTATA

Even saying the word frittata makes me smile. I'm not sure why, but frittatas have always made me think of fun, perhaps because they're typically served at Sunday brunches or while dining at elegant French cafés with friends. They're also the ideal vehicle for protein and veggies: this Superhuman Breakfast Frittata can be eaten for breakfast, lunch or dinner, and it ALWAYS hits the spot. I'll typically make this for brunch on a relaxed weekend morning and try to keep some leftovers (if I can stop my hubby from eating it all!) for a meal or two on Monday or Tuesday.

MAKES 4–6 SERVINGS

10–12 large eggs, separated

1 teaspoon sea salt

¼ teaspoon freshly ground black pepper

2 tablespoons coconut oil

2 garlic cloves, crushed

1 onion, diced

1 sweet potato, very finely diced or grated

2 or 3 kale leaves, deveined and chopped, or 60–90g baby spinach or rocket

1 tablespoon Italian seasoning, or 5g chopped fresh herbs

Sprinkle of grated raw goats' cheese, crumbled soft goats' cheese or feta (optional)

1 Preheat the oven to 180°C/gas mark 4.

2 Beat the egg whites in a medium bowl until frothy. Whisk in the egg yolks to combine. Add the sea salt and pepper; stir and set aside.

3 In a 25cm non-stick ovenproof frying pan (ideally cast iron), melt the coconut oil on a medium heat.

4 Add the garlic, onion and sweet potato and season with sea salt and pepper.

5 Toss to coat the veggies in the oil and cook until you can almost stab through the sweet potato with a fork. Add your greens and sauté for a further 2 minutes.

6 Pour in the egg mixture so that the vegetables and eggs are distributed evenly and add the Italian seasoning or herbs.

7 Let everything cook undisturbed for 5–7 minutes, or until the edges are set and slightly brown and the center is slightly wobbly when you shake the pan.

8 Put the pan in the oven and cook for another 5–7 minutes, until the frittata has set completely. If using the cheese, add it during the last 2 minutes of cooking.

9 Take the frittata out of the oven and allow it to cool in the pan for 5 minutes..

10 Slice it into wedges to serve.

OVERNIGHT OATS

So many mornings do not go as we imagine. We get a rushed, late start or kids, partners and phones get in the way. Finally dressed and already running late, we now have ZERO time for breakfast. Enter Overnight Oats. If you know your mornings can be hectic, throw some oats, a milk alternative and a few other fun ingredients into a jar and leave them in the fridge overnight. Now you've got a portable breakfast for you and the kids! You can make a few jars at a time and keep them in the fridge for those grab-and-go mornings. Experiment with your add-ins too! What wouldn't be delicious in here?

MAKES 1 SERVING

40g rolled oats

240ml Alternative Milk (see page 72)

Pinch of sea salt

1 tablespoon protein powder of choice (optional)

Sweetener of choice: stevia, coconut sugar, maple syrup, or honey

MIX-INS: Nut butter, cocoa or raw cacao powder, no-sugar-added jam, shredded coconut, smashed fruit, ground flax meal, chia seeds, cinnamon

1 Combine the oats, alternative milk and salt in a bowl or jar. Cover and refrigerate overnight.

2 In the morning, remove from the fridge. Add protein powder, sweetener and additional mix-ins if you like, then eat! If you prefer your oats warm, you can gently heat them in a pan on the hob before eating.

AMARANTH PORRIDGE

Love a warm bowl of goodness first thing in the morning? This simple, but satisfying, porridge will definitely hit the spot. Rich and creamy, it's the perfect platform for your favourite mix-ins – anything from almond butter to cacao, goji berries and shredded coconut flakes can work in here. This breakfast also works if you're eating it at room temperature, just in case you need to pack your meal to go. Plus, amaranth is a powerful little seed that's naturally anti-inflammatory, a great source of fibre and a complete protein. It even has Lysine, the rare amino acid that helps the body absorb calcium, build muscle and produce energy. Any non-dairy milk can be substituted for the coconut milk.

MAKES 2 SERVINGS

100g amaranth

475ml coconut milk (store-bought without carrageenan) or Alternative Milk (see page 72)

¼ teaspoon sea salt

Mix-ins and sweetener of choice

1 Put the amaranth, coconut milk and salt in a small saucepan and bring to the boil.

2 Simmer for 20–30 minutes, until the amaranth is soft and has reached a porridge-like consistency.

3 Top with ingredients of your choice.

APPLE CHIA 'CEREAL'

'I'm on board, Robyn', you say. 'But I'm sorry, you will never keep me away from my cereal.' This recipe was created especially with you in mind. Again, it began with a simple kitchen experiment: could I satisfy my cereal lovers and still give them something simple, gut friendly and packed with nutrition? With more than 15 grams of easy-to-absorb fibre, thanks to the apple and chia seeds, the answer is a very delicious yes.

MAKES 1 SERVING

2 tablespoons chia seeds

120ml Alternative Milk (see page 72)

2 or 3 drops vanilla stevia

Pinch of sea salt

¼ teaspoon spirulina (fun 'green milk', optional)

1 small apple with skin, chopped

1 teaspoon ground cinnamon, or more to taste

1–2 tablespoons finely chopped walnuts

1 tablespoon grated unsweetened coconut

1 Stir together the chia seeds, milk, stevia, salt and spirulina (if using) in a bowl. Put them in the refrigerator to set, about 10 minutes.

2 Layer a bowl or to-go container with the apple, cinnamon and walnuts.

3 Once the chia mixture has set, stir and taste; add more stevia if necessary.

4 Stir the apples into the chia mix and finish with the coconut and more cinnamon, if desired.

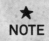

★ NOTE

The chia mix can be made the night before. The entire dish can also be prepared the night before as long as you don't mind slightly brown apples that are a little softer in texture.

EGGS AND OATS

Are you a morning warm oats lover? Here's a simple way to increase the protein and satisfaction in your breakfast bowl. The addition of eggs also makes the oats nice and fluffy. You'll barely notice they're there!

MAKES 1–2 SERVINGS

120ml water

120ml Alternative Milk(see page 72)

⅛ teaspoon of sea salt, more to taste

40g rolled oats

2 eggs

Spices of your choice

1 teaspoon ground chia or flax seeds

(optional)

1 Heat the water and alternative milk in a saucepan until boiling.

2 Add the sea salt and oats. Reduce to a simmer.

3 In a bowl, scramble the eggs and add them to the oats stirring constantly. Allow the egg/oat combo to cook until the oats are soft, about 5–15 minutes depending on the type of oats used.

4 Season with spices of choice, chia or flax seeds, if using, and additional salt if needed (you can go sweet or savoury!) and serve.

SWEET CINNAMON SCRAMBLE

Craving something sweet for breakfast but still want your power-packed eggs? This slightly kooky egg dish has got you covered. I created this in my kitchen as I was standing there thinking, how would cinnamon be with eggs? The answer? It's delicious!

MAKES 1 SERVING

2 teaspoons coconut oil

1 carrot, grated

2 eggs

1 teaspoon vanilla extract

Small handful of baby spinach (optional)

Sea salt and freshly ground pepper, to

taste

½ teaspoon cinnamon, or more to taste

1 Heat coconut oil and grated carrot in a sauté pan over medium heat.

2 Beat the eggs and vanilla extract in a small bowl.

3 Once the carrots begin to soften, about 2 minutes, add the eggs and baby spinach, if using.

4 Season with sea salt, pepper and cinnamon and scramble the mixture while cooking through. Once the eggs are cooked to your liking, sprinkle with additional cinnamon and serve.

CHIA CAKES

Ohhh, do I love these little cakes. Awesome as breakfast and great for a snack, they feel decadent and FUN to eat. Serve them with Sweet Cinnamon Sauce or Nut Butter Sauce (see recipes below) or experiment with your own toppings, snap a pic and tag me on social media with #GoWithYourGutBook @robynyoukilis!

MAKES 1 SERVING

1 banana or 1 small sweet potato, peeled and steamed until very soft

1 or 2 eggs, depending on size of banana or sweet potato used

1 tablespoon chia seeds

⅛ teaspoon sea salt

1 teaspoon coconut flour, if needed

1 tablespoon butter, coconut oil or ghee

NOTE

These pancakes do best with a double-utensil flip since they are less sturdy than traditional pancakes.

1 Mash the banana or sweet potato with the back of a fork until broken up. You can also use a blender or food processor.

2 Stir in the eggs, chia seeds and sea salt and mix until thoroughly combined.

3 Allow the mixture to sit at room temperature, ideally for 5 minutes. If the batter looks too thin, add the coconut flour and mix.

4 Place a 25cm frying pan over a medium heat. Add the butter, coconut oil or ghee and heat until it melts.

5 Place about 60ml of batter in the pan to form a pancake. When the edges start to turn white, the pancake is ready to flip. Fry it on the other side until cooked through, then serve immediately with toppings. Repeat with the remaining batter.

SWEET CINNAMON SAUCE

2 tablespoons yogurt (goat's or ewe's milk)

1 tablespoon non-dairy milk

⅛ teaspoon ground cinnamon

1 drop stevia or vanilla stevia (optional)

Pinch of sea salt

Mix all the ingredients in a bowl and serve immediately.

NUT BUTTER SAUCE

1 tablespoon nut butter

2 tablespoons non-dairy milk

1 drop stevia (optional)

Mix all the ingredients in a bowl and serve immediately.

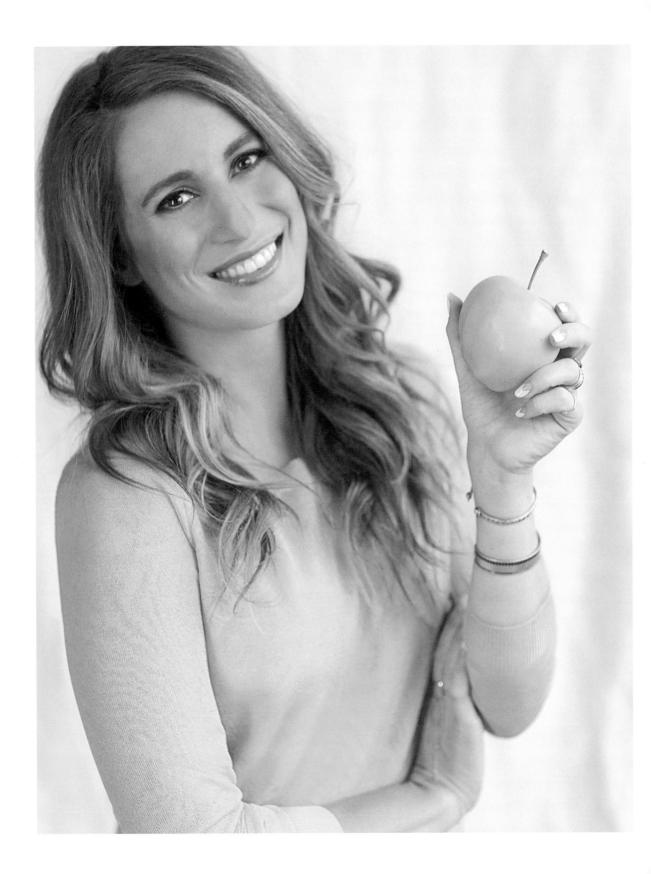

CHAPTER 2

CHEW

The number one question I get asked by my audience is, 'What's the most important thing I can do right now to feel better, be healthier and lose weight?' My answer is always the same:

You need to learn how to start chewing your food.

If you stop to think about it, has anyone ever taught you HOW to eat? Think back to your childhood. Aside from 'Don't talk with your mouth full', 'Finish your veggies' and 'Keep your elbows off the table', did anyone ever say, 'THIS is how you chew and how many bites per mouthful you need in order to properly digest what you are putting into your belly?' Did they explain that this is something you will do every single day for the rest of your life? That you must chew, until liquid, always, before you swallow? This little matter of chewing your food is the likely culprit behind most common digestive issues.

NEWS FLASH: YOUR STOMACH DOESN'T HAVE TEETH

I constantly remind my community, 'Your stomach doesn't have teeth', so don't expect it to do your chewing for you!

I'm here to get you to practise chewing more. Depending on the food, aim to chew anywhere from 20 to 50 times with each mouthful. Some monks chew to 100 (I haven't actually met any of these monks, but I would like to!).

Chewing is the best (and totally free!) practice to give your brain enough time to catch up with your belly. It takes at least 20 minutes for our body to process that it's eaten anything and most of us finish a very large meal in less time than that. If you do the maths, you'll realise you aren't giving your body a chance to signal that it's had enough before you clean your plate.

Food that cannot be digested (i.e. anything you swallow that isn't chewed thoroughly), is not necessarily eliminated, but can turn into debris in the body and cause inflammation. Essentially, you are leaving too many windows open on your computer, confusing and over-tasking it, and instead of uploading the video immediately, your body has to push through that upload signal. This will sound so foreign – and you may not realise how far you probably are from doing this and how strange it will feel at first – but you want to chew your food until it is completely transformed from solid to mush. Most of us are not remotely used to what this feels like inside our mouths. It took me at least 2 years of determined practice and patience before I felt I was doing this unconsciously. I still sometimes catch myself swallowing after five chews. I have to check myself when I'm feeling impatient and want to rebel.

This applies to everyone – whether you're eating your lunch at your desk or dining al fresco on your yacht in Tahiti. You could be from any culture with any type of cuisine from anywhere on the globe; everyone needs to chew their food, allowing the saliva that was designed to work on our food to do its job.

I can't think of better proof of the effect chewing has on the entire body than the story of what inspired Lino Stanchich, to write the book *Power Eating Program: You Are How You Eat*. In 1943, Stanchich's father, Antonio, was in a concentration camp in Germany, and in spite of being forced into hard labour, he was given very little to eat and drink. He witnessed many of his fellow prisoners die every day from starvation. In the frigid weather, Antonio began a habit that would save his life. Lino says in his book:

When my father was thirsty, he kept the cold water in his mouth to warm it and intuitively 'chewed' it for a while, 10 to 15 times, before swallowing. One day, when the water was especially cold, he chewed it 50 times! And he discovered something that would save his life.

Aside from quenching his thirst, the water actually seemed to give him energy. At first he felt it must be his imagination. Eventually he realised that chewing water 50 times or more did indeed give him more energy. Puzzled, he asked himself how plain water could impart

such a miracle. It took 40 years to clarify this mystery.

My father experimented by chewing his food 50 times a mouthful. Then he tried 75, 100, 150, 200, even up to 300 times or more. He determined that the magical minimum number of chews was 150 and the more he chewed, the more energy he had. The morning and noon meals were restricted in time, but the evening meal was not. In the evening he could chew water as much as he liked.

My father's technique was simple: put one tablespoon of food, either liquid or solid, in the mouth and count your chews. Most of his friends scoffed at his discovery. But two men became interested in these experiments and joined my father in his chewing sessions. Comparing notes, they both concluded that this technique did give them more energy. And they also felt warmer and less hungry.

In 1945, after two years in the concentration camp, the prisoners were liberated by the U.S. Army. In time, my father, skinny but alive, came home to us in Fiume-Rijeka, formerly part of Italy, now Yugoslavia. Of his crew of 32 from the concentration camp, only three survived: my

tip

Soups and smoothies need chewing too! Try and allow those foods to have a little time in your mouth before swallowing as they too benefit from the enzymes in your saliva.

IT'S TIME TO START TAKING OUR TIME WITH FOOD. RELAX AND ENJOY AND... CRUNCH AWAY!

father, and the two men who joined him in his practice of chewing.

The following year, when I was 14, while on a family picnic, my father told me of his experience. He attributed his survival exclusively to chewing. He gave me some important advice, saying: 'If you are ever weak, cold or sick, chew each mouthful 150 times or more'. I never forgot those words, even though we had plenty of food and I was in good health.

What chewing does is truly amazing. When you let your mouth do the work it was designed for, the rest of your body is able to receive the minerals and nutrients from what you have eaten and to properly utilise its contents. Contrary to what you might imagine, it is not the job of your belly (intestines, etc.) to break down food. Swallowing whole or poorly chewed bites of food sets off a disastrous chain of events.

Your body goes into crisis management mode. Organs that are normally performing necessary functions to maintain homeostasis in your body are forced to begrudgingly assist in digesting. They respond with inflammation. They talk

back with farts, belches, bloating, acid reflux and heartburn!

Just as with cortisol, inflammation itself is not a bad thing. It is an imbalanced inflammatory response that causes issues. I'll say it again: we strive to help our bodies work the way they are designed to instead of forcing them to react to crisis or extremity. Inflammation is designed to help your body fight infection. But when the bacteria your body is trying to fight, or the virus it is acting to eliminate is not there, your body is attacking itself. That's the inflammatory reaction we don't want to happen. The more confusion and debris, the bigger the chance this is going to happen.

It's time to start taking our time with food. Relax and enjoy and ... crunch away! My 21-day Chewing Challenge will put you on the right path.

★

THE 21-DAY CHEWING CHALLENGE

I created a 21-day Chewing Challenge to help you build your chewing habit.

For 21 days, you'll receive daily emails, recipes, and inspiration to help make this new practice fun and doable. Sign up at www.robynyoukilis.com/gutbookbonuses.

For added inspiration, here's a success story from one of my amazing clients who gave this a try:

I've struggled with digestion for as long as I can remember. For the last three to four years, my constipation got so bad that I would go 10 days without a trip to the bathroom. In a typical week, I'd go two or three times. I've been on a health journey since finding out I was intolerant to dairy in 2010. I found a naturopath and went the more natural route with probiotics, HCL and a gluten-free diet. I've spent thousands of dollars on testing for vitamin and mineral deficiencies, hormone imbalances, SIBO and food intolerances. While the results were super interesting and even game changing for reasons other than digestion, nothing seemed to help with constipation.

After thousands more dollars spent on follow-up appointments and supplements to fix what we found, I still wasn't pooping. Fast-forward 6 months to when I met you and you told me about the 21-day Chewing Challenge. All I heard was 'If you are not pooping, you need to start chewing,' and I was in! I started the challenge and noticed an improvement in 48 hours. Of the 21 days, I pooped 18! I'd call that revolutionary and it was SO simple... yet not always easy. Every time I have a mouthful of food, I think, 'is this mush? Could I chew a few more times before swallowing?'

Additionally, the challenge has changed my relationship with food. So many foods that I was eating, I found I didn't really like. If I don't want to chew it, I am not eating it anymore. I realized that more often than not, I was eating for pleasure/stimulation/distraction, rather than health and sustenance. It's a journey and I have a long way to go, but just being aware of how quickly I'm swallowing and how food feels in my mouth is a huge improvement in my overall health. I am so grateful to have met you and to have this tool to help me along the way. Thank you for putting this out into the world!

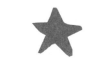

CHEW RECIPES

Perfect for practising your new chewing habit, this fresh approach to eating more raw vegetables for snack time will really give you something to crunch on.

Spiced Raw Veggies –
Sweet and Spicy Seasoning or
Mexican Seasoning
Jicama Chips –
Cinnamon Sprinkle or
Lime and Sea Salt

SPICED RAW VEGGIES

Girl, if you're going to get your raw veggie on, you've got to spice them up. Not only do the spices naturally aid in the digestive process, they're also delicious and make you much more likely to opt for raw veggies when you're just looking for something to munch on in the afternoon.

FOR EACH SERVING:

300–400g chopped raw veggies of choice – carrots, celery, cucumbers, etc.
Some fun different veggie suggestions: kohlrabi, jicama, celeriac, green beans, broccoli stalks

SWEET AND SPICY SEASONING

1 teaspoon curry powder

1 teaspoon ground cinnamon

Pinch of sea salt

Pinch of cayenne pepper

MEXICAN SEASONING

1 teaspoon ground cumin

¼ teaspoon cayenne pepper

¼ - ½ teaspoon chilli powder (optional)

1 tablespoon lime juice

¼ teaspoon sea salt

Choose your seasoning variation, Sweet and Spicy or Mexican, combine all the ingredients in a small bowl and toss together until the veggies are coated in spices. Serve immediately.

tip

You'll want to choose glass storage and to-go containers as much as possible over plastic. Plastic usually contains BPA that can leach from containers and into your food. Food stored in glass containers also tastes better and stores better (and easily goes from fridge to oven to table).

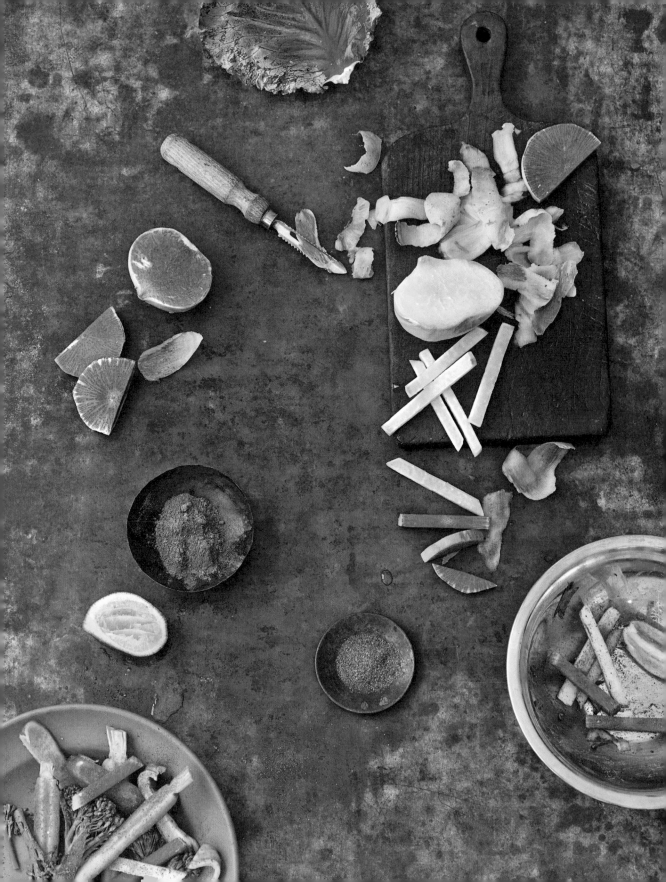

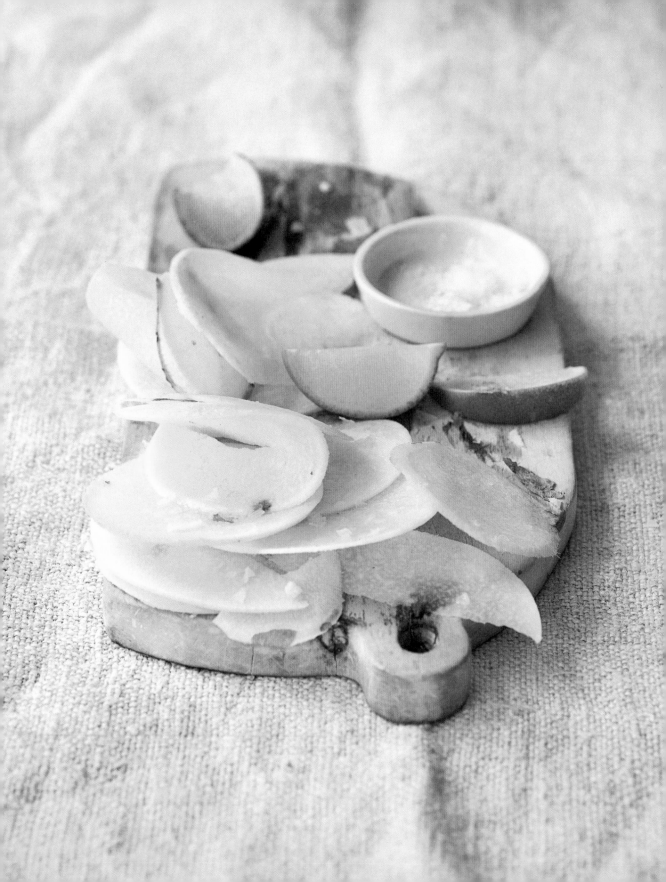

JICAMA CHIPS

Typically relegated to gigantic Mexican BBQ-style salads, jicama deserves its own time in the spotlight. A perfect Go With Your Gut *food, it's rich in pre-biotic fibre (which promotes healthy gut flora), filled with water, light, crunchy and takes on the flavours of any kind of seasoning your little heart desires. If you can't find jicama, kohlrabi makes a wonderful substitute.*

FOR EACH SERVING:

1 medium jicama, peeled and cut into very thin slices with a mandolin or sticks with a knife

CINNAMON SPRINKLE

2 teaspoons ground cinnamon

Pinch of sea salt

LIME AND SEA SALT

Juice of ½ lime

2 pinches of sea salt

Sprinkle the jicama with the toppings of your choice. Store in the fridge for up to 3 days.

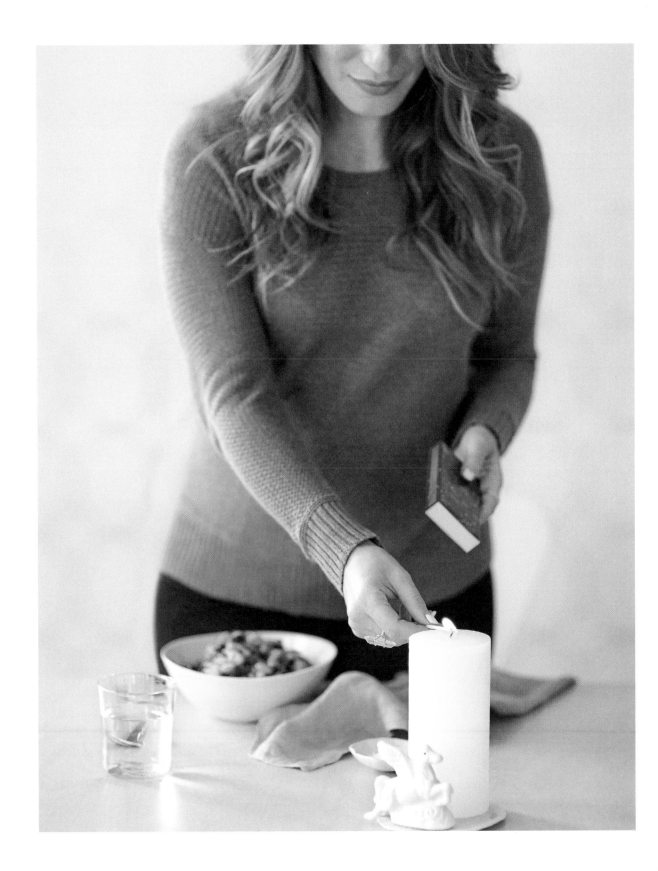

CHAPTER 3

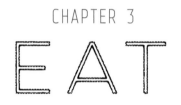

Somewhere along the line, many of us develop poor eating habits: emotional eating, stress eating, mindless eating. Over time, these habits cause issues such as moodiness, stomach aches and excess weight. Also, many people end up taking over-the-counter meds such as Gaviscon and Zantac to treat the body's reaction to mindless overeating. These medications may have long-term consequences on your digestive system, especially when used frequently. I don't advocate any of these types of 'solutions'; they have negative side effects and can confuse and muddy our ability to understand what's really going on in our bodies. Most importantly, most of these issues can be resolved without popping a pill.

For most of us, bad eating habits become a never-ending cycle of negative emotions that take up a huge amount of mental space. It goes like this; you hate yourself because you know you should be eating better, and the fact that you're not is your fault. You don't think you have the willpower or strength to follow through on what you plan to do. So, you feel guilty, and in order to resolve that guilt, you turn to cookies or a packet of crisps.

But here's the truth: lack of willpower is not the reason why you eat this way. The Food and Brand Lab is a research department at Cornell University that examines all the different elements that affect how much and which foods we eat. Their research is astounding. For instance, do you know that the colour of your plate matters? It does! (Hint: choose soothing colours like blue over yellow, as bright warm colours naturally stimulate appetite.) Cornell has tons of such studies, which all support the fact that our environment has a crazy amount of power over our eating habits. Another example: if a friend says something that stresses you out at dinner, you're more likely to order macaroni cheese than opt for veggies and fish. When you consider the results of these studies, you might rethink those bad habits you've developed over time. They're definitely not all your fault! So let's end the blame game. It. Stops. Right. Here. OK?

In one of those classic *Sex and the City* scenes that is imprinted in my brain, I fell in love with the image of Carrie Bradshaw standing in the kitchen of her stylish apartment eating crackers with jam (a college favourite of mine) as she flipped through fashion magazines, something she described as 'Secret Single Behavior'. It seemed so glamorous to me; it was such a marker of the independent, cool, city girl. However, this is what we do, us on-the-go-gals: we stand and eat with one hand while texting with the other. Maybe you feel busy and important and in-demand (and you are!) when that phone lights up every minute, but let's take a second to be present with ourselves and, of course, our food.

HOW TO: MINDFUL EATING

So what to do? First, going over what we learnt in the last chapter, chew. Chew until your food is mush or liquid, and eat more slowly. Use your new chewing habit to slow it all down – the whole experience.

Next, it's time to turn off the TV. It is way harder to know when you are full and satiated if you are wildly distracted as you eat (not to mention all the appetite-stimulating commercials and shows you wind up watching). As I share in the 21-day Chewing Challenge, when you eat with distractions, you wind up feeling as if you never ate at all. You tend to eat much faster and chew less.

Practising mindful eating is the best way to change those habits that no longer serve you, and to counteract the subconscious factors that get in the way of achieving your health and wellness goals. I know that the sheer mention of mindful eating usually results in an eye roll and probably a sigh. I thought that way too, before I learned what mindful eating truly was. After I became a health coach, I used to think I ate mindfully. I was wrong.

The first time I really 'got' mindful eating, I was at a retreat at the Kripaul Center for Yoga and Health in Massachusetts, taking one of my continuing education programmes for nutrition professionals. After I completed my own eye rolls and got to work, I realised how

transformative an experience mindful eating can be. The teacher had us each take one almond in our hands. She instructed us to really look at it. What did we notice? How did it smell? How much could we observe before taking our first bites? I quickly realised how beautiful nature's foods are. The striations in the almond, the lovely light brown colour; this one little almond was a little piece of art.

Next, we tasted. Anything we noticed there? Was it smooth? Rough? How exactly could we describe the texture? And then, finally, we chewed. What flavours did we immediately notice? What flavours did we notice after it was completely chewed until liquid? Were they different from what we noticed at first? It blew me away how sweet the almond tasted the more I chewed – something I had never really noticed before. It had taken me 10 minutes to eat one almond. It was an experience I'll never forget. The more I incorporated mindful eating into my routine in a natural, innate way, the easier it was for me to be happy and satisfied with so much less. And because I was eating less food, I was beginning to lose weight without even realising it!

GUT GUIDELINES

GUT GUIDELINE #1

Try to eat with minimal distractions. I know that this might seem boring, but we all know that eating while watching a TV show or endlessly scrolling our social media feeds, finishing our meal absorbed in the show or photo stream, ends with us thinking 'now what can I eat?' What's worse, you keep eating without noticing those body signals of fullness or discomfort.

Every slow meal you eat mindfully, with just music on or a friend eating with you, gets rid of the idea that you 'should' eat more food or that you need to keep munching while you're doing something else. Instead, you'll be focused on your food and the complete experience of eating – texture, taste, smell, how the food makes you feel and more. And I don't expect you to practise this at every meal, every moment of the day. Just start with one meal or snack and baby-step your way up from there.

GUT GUIDELINE #2

Aim to be no longer hungry instead of full. I like to imagine my stomach as a container that I might mix a homemade salad dressing in. I add all the ingredients, but I have to be careful not to add too much because there needs to be some room for me to shake the container and emulsify everything together. Your stomach operates the same way – it needs a little room for what you've eaten to mix and properly digest.

That's why I advise my *Go With Your Gut* Gals to gain a sense of being 'no longer hungry' instead of striving to be full all the time. Personally, I've found that when I'm concerned with being 'full', eating is really about something (or someone) else that's not satisfying me. It's about a feeling that I'm trying to numb out by eating.

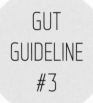

GUT GUIDELINE #3

Smaller plates, smaller bowls, smaller everything! This is a trick research taught me, and it's really simple. The same amount of food on a smaller plate looks larger to your eye – thus, you eat less. Use your salad or medium-sized plates instead of gigantic dinner plates. Use your smaller bowls. It's an easy swap, a great opportunity to refresh your kitchen style, and has huge effects on how much food you eat at a meal.

You're not always going to be perfect. In fact, let's just toss that word out of the window right now. You might still binge on crisps and guacamole (it's just soo delicious; I get it). It's okay; we've all been there. And stop with the scales – they'll drive you crazy. Screw focusing on weight loss; don't worry about the number, because the natural fluctuations we all have – down two pounds one day, up three the next – raises your stress, messes with your hormones and puts you right back on the guilt cycle that's made you unhappy and/or frustrated. Let's all just understand right now that your weight will always fluctuate. And it's completely okay. What's not okay is living a lifetime with a 'goal weight' your body doesn't agree with. Let's toss that 'goal weight' right out along with the scales.

Let's be as kind to ourselves as we would be to others; remember to focus on all the amazing things we are doing and those habits will naturally change one by one. And so will your beautiful body.

EAT RECIPES

This section was created just for my 'Give me the darn recipe and tell me exactly what to do' peeps! I love experimenting in the kitchen; it's how these recipes were created – but sometimes we want a single clear recipe that makes a complete meal. A lot of these dishes are perfect to make in double batches, either for company or to store in the fridge and eat throughout the week. They're part of this chapter because they encompass everything Eat is about! Feed your body whole, real, natural foods in a satisfying form and take-aways will suddenly start to seem a lot less appealing.

Kabocha Squash and Kale Tacos
Happy Joes
Perfect Detox Salad
Moroccan-Spiced Kale Salad
Stuffed Acorn Squash
Burger - Fish, Turkey, Chicken, Black Bean
Cauliflower Rice
Classic Curry
Shepherd's Pie

KABOCHA SQUASH
AND KALE TACOS

The inspiration for this dish came from a little vegan café near my apartment. When that restaurant sadly closed, I knew I had to recreate the recipe at home. They used butternut squash, which works nicely, but I roast kabocha more often and love its denseness. I frequently make this dish for company and people rave over it. The flavours are great, it's easy to throw together and friends can customise their toppings. Plus, you'll easily cover the special needs of your vegan, vegetarian and gluten-free and/or dairy-free friends. Sometimes I'll eat the combo in a corn or sprouted grain tortilla or create a 'bowl' with quinoa, salad greens or both. Add some freshly chopped tomatoes, additional coriander, sliced avocado and a squeeze of lime for a truly delectable dish.

MAKES 4 SERVINGS

1 kabocha or butternut squash (see Note), washed, dried, halved lengthways and seeds scooped out

3–4 tablespoons melted coconut oil

Sea salt and freshly ground black pepper

8 × 15cm tortillas

Garlicky Restaurant-style Greens (page 90)

TOPPINGS

Black beans (fresh or canned), drained and rinsed well

Sprinkle of Mexican-style seasoning

Chopped fresh tomatoes

Avocado slices

Chopped fresh coriander

Grated cheese (I suggest hard goats' cheese)

Coriander Yogurt Dressing (see page 171)

Lime wedges

1 Preheat the oven to 220°C/gas mark 7.

2 Cut the squash crossways in thin slices (do your best!).

3 Place them on a baking tray and coat with the coconut oil. Season generously with salt and pepper.

4 Bake for 20 minutes. Turn the slices over and test for doneness by poking with a fork (if it's soft enough to eat, taste for seasoning and add more salt if needed).

5 Add additional cooking time, probably another 10–20 minutes, depending on the thickness of the slices. Poke and taste again!

6 Warm the tortillas one by one in a frying pan. Keep them warm by wrapping the heated tortillas on a plate with a clean tea towel.

7 In a small pan, warm the black beans and stir in a sprinkle of Mexican seasoning.

8 Fill each tortilla with the greens, squash, beans and desired toppings.

★
NOTE

You may substitute fresh or frozen cubed organic butternut squash for a shortcut!

HAPPY JOES

As a kid, I loooooved Sloppy Joes (minced beef served in a hamburger bun). Ours was a pretty healthy household, though, and my mum would rarely make anything that crossed into the junk-food category. So, naturally, that's all I wanted. I remember waiting for the school canteen to serve this food like it was my birthday! Here, I've taken the flavours and idea of a Sloppy Joe, but made it easy to digest and healthy. This recipe is great served over Cauliflower Rice (see page 58), on a mashed or baked sweet potato, with your favourite salad or, best of all, in my Shepherd's Pie (see page 61).

MAKES 4–6 SERVINGS

1 tablespoon olive oil or coconut oil

1 medium yellow onion, finely diced

2 garlic cloves, chopped or crushed

450g protein (minced beef or turkey, cooked lentils or crumbled tempeh all work great)

1–2 teaspoons chilli powder

2 teaspoons dried oregano

1 teaspoon sea salt

55g tomato purée

1 × 230g can chopped tomatoes

1 tablespoon Dijon mustard

Garnishes: toasted flaked almonds, chopped fresh coriander and/or parsley

1 Heat the oil in a large pan over a medium–low heat. Sauté the onion for about 10 minutes, until translucent.

2 Add the garlic and sauté for 1 more minute.

3 Add protein of choice, chilli powder, oregano and salt and stir.

4 Add the tomato purée, chopped tomatoes and mustard; stir and cook for 5 minutes.

5 Add up to 450ml water as needed to create a sauce; stir and cook for another 5 minutes, until the protein is cooked through. Serve immediately, with garnishes.

tip

If you have kids that love sweet foods, add 1 tablespoon of maple syrup in Step 4!

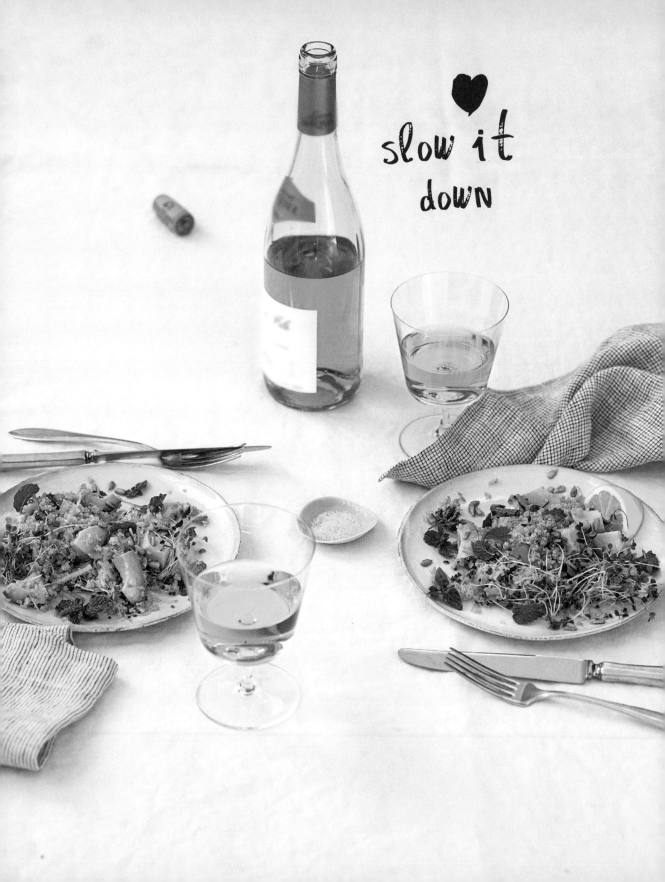

slow it
down

PERFECT DETOX SALAD

Since L.A. is where Scott and I began dating, it holds a special place in our hearts. We spend months at a time there throughout the year, swapping apartments so that we can do the activities and see the people we love. During one of our L.A. stints, I created this recipe from ingredients I purchased at the local farmers' market. From the perfectly ripe avocados to the Meyer lemons, it is the perfect Cali livin' dish. Light, fresh and bright, it's totally moreish and also very, very good for you. If I want a green salad option for lunch, I'll swap the quinoa for salad greens. Be sure to include the mint and tons of lemon juice, preferably from Meyer lemons, if you can find them – they really make this salad spectacular.

MAKES 2 TO 4 SERVINGS

175g uncooked quinoa (or 200g salad greens)

1 daikon radish, grated

2 carrots, grated

20–35g mix of micro greens and/or sprouts
of any kind

½ bunch fresh mint leaves, roughly chopped
or torn

1 avocado, diced

Handful of raw sunflower seeds

Juice of 1 lemon, preferably Meyer

2 tablespoons extra-virgin olive oil

Sea salt and freshly ground black pepper,
to taste

⅛ teaspoon cayenne pepper

1 Cook the quinoa according to the instructions on page 167. Drain and use it warm or refrigerate it until cold, depending on your preference.

2 To make the salad, combine all the ingredients thoroughly and serve immediately!

tip

I eat minimal grains, while my hubby eats maximum grains. So how do we get along when it comes to dinnertime? Simple: about twice a week I'll throw either quinoa or millet (or a mix of the two!) into the rice cooker for him, 'set it and forget it' style. I chose those as the main grains featured in this book because they are the easiest to digest, naturally gluten-free, alkalising and high in protein. You can add these grains to almost any of the star dishes for an extra-filling meal. The directions to make them can be found on page 167.

MOROCCAN-SPICED KALE SALAD

Probably my most famous recipe, this salad was featured online as the kale salad Anderson Cooper said he'd love to try. Thousands of website hits and a million Moroccan-Spiced Kale Salads later, I knew you guys had to have this recipe. Kale, often considered the godfather of all leafy greens, is packed with nutrients your body loves. Rich in vitamins A, C, E and K, calcium, magnesium and iron, it's one of the best greens you can go with.

MAKES 2–4 SERVINGS

1 bunch Tuscan kale (sometimes referred to as dino or lacinato kale), ribs removed and leaves roughly chopped (or use any other variety of kale)

2 tablespoons extra-virgin olive oil

Sea salt

Juice of ½ lemon

1 teaspoon ground cumin

1 teaspoon ground turmeric

1 medium carrot, peeled and finely grated

½ crisp apple, peeled, cored and finely chopped

40g sultanas (or raisins)

25g flaked almonds

3 tablespoons pitted oil-cured olives (about 9), halved

2 tablespoons hemp seeds (optional)

Freshly ground black pepper

1 In a medium bowl, combine the kale with the olive oil. Sprinkle with sea salt. Using your hands, massage the kale until the oil coats the leaves and they begin to wilt, about 1–2 minutes.

2 In a small bowl, whisk the lemon juice with the cumin and turmeric. Add the mixture to the kale and toss the leaves until well combined.

3 Add the carrot, apple, sultanas, almonds, olives and hemp seeds, if using; toss until just combined. Season with more salt and some pepper. Let the salad rest for 5–10 minutes, then serve.

tip

'Did you just tell me to "massage" a vegetable?' Yep! Massaging 'tougher' and more fibrous greens such as kale (literally rubbing them back and forth in your hands until they wilt), helps to soften the greens, making them more enjoyable to eat raw and easier to digest.

STUFFED ACORN SQUASH

I love a good all-in-one-dish kind of meal like this Stuffed Acorn Squash. You can make the stuffing ahead of time and then bake the squashes when you're ready to serve, or prep and pop them in the oven while you entertain friends over appetizers. Squash is what I like to call a 'super starch'. It's anti-inflammatory and high in antioxidants, magnesium, potassium, vitamin C and fibre. You can make this dish grain-free by simply omitting the grains and adding some extra veggies or beans. If you include grains, quinoa works beautifully, or try a fun new grain, kaniwah! Similar to quinoa, kaniwah is a tiny seed (about half the size of quinoa) that has many of the same nutritional properties, like being high in fiber and protein!

MAKES 4–6 SERVINGS

2 small acorn squashes, halved and seeded

Coconut oil

Sea salt and freshly ground black pepper

2 garlic cloves, crushed

1 yellow onion, finely diced

2 courgettes, finely diced

100g chickpeas, chopped (optional)

40g chopped fresh mushrooms

2 tablespoons finely chopped fresh sage

2 tablespoons fresh thyme

375–550g cooked quinoa or kaniwah (see page 167)

25g chopped pistachio nuts (pine nuts work well too)

Chilli flakes

Small handful of chopped fresh parsley

Sprinkle of cheese (optional, but I love raw goats' cheese or crumbled feta)

1 Preheat the oven to 220°C/gas mark 7.

2 Coat the squash halves with coconut oil and season with sea salt and pepper (if serving a large party or as a side dish you can cut the halves into quarters).

3 Roast them cut-side down on a baking sheet until fork-soft, about 25–40 minutes depending on your oven.

4 While the squash is roasting, sauté the garlic and onions in a large frying pan over medium heat in 1–2 tablespoons of coconut oil until everything begins to soften, about 3–4 minutes.

5 Add the courgettes, chickpeas, mushrooms, sage and thyme and continue to cook until everything is softened and brown, about 5–10 minutes depending on thickness and types of vegetables used.

6 Fold together the sautéed vegetables, cooked grains, pistachios, chilli flakes and most of the parsley. Add sea salt, pepper and a drizzle of oil, if needed.

7 Fill the squash halves with stuffing and top with cheese, if using. Place in the oven or under a grill until the filling has browned a bit or the cheese has fully melted. Serve immediately.

tip

If you have picky eaters in your family, create the simplest version for the table and offer the optional add-ins or dressings and sauces on the side.

BURGER
FISH, TURKEY, CHICKEN, BLACK BEAN

Nothing beats a good burger. While I was thinking about and researching what kind of burger I wanted to include in this book, this recipe came to me via a dear friend. She texted me immediately after making it, exclaiming how easy and delicious these burgers were, and telling me that I must include them in my book! From fashion to food, her taste is impeccable, so I knew I had to take her seriously. The original recipe had panko breadcrumbs, but when I got in the kitchen I immediately thought: desiccated coconut! Light and fluffy and nutritionally rich coconut plus a few additional healthy tweaks and voilà! – a simple and delicious burger recipe that works with any protein. I suggest you master this one immediately.

MAKES 4 SERVINGS

450g minced chicken, turkey or beef
or fish or 2 × 400g cans black beans, drained
and rinsed

1 egg white, beaten

75g desiccated unsweetened coconut

1 tablespoon garlic powder

1 tablespoon chopped dried onion flakes
(these also make a great crunchy salad
topping!)

60ml tamari or coconut aminos

1–2 tablespoons coconut oil

Coriander Yogurt Dressing, to serve

★
NOTES

*You can also bake these in the oven at 180°C/
gas mark 4 until cooked through to your liking.*

*The bean burgers can be a bit crumbly when
serving, but they're still delicious!*

1 If using beans, grind them in a food processor until crumbly. If using fish, you can ask your fishmonger to grind for you or grind at home using same process as beans. If you don't have a food processor, you can chop beans or fish finely with a knife.

2 Mix the protein together in a large bowl with the remaining ingredients and shape into four large patties or six mini patties.

3 Add the oil to your frying pan and cook the burgers over medium heat until golden brown on the bottom, 3–6 minutes depending on protein. Flip the burgers over.

4 Reduce the heat to low and cook for another 5 minutes, until brown or crisp. Serve immediately with traditional burger toppings, on top of a salad or in a lettuce wrap. I love topping them with the Coriander Yogurt Dressing on page 171.

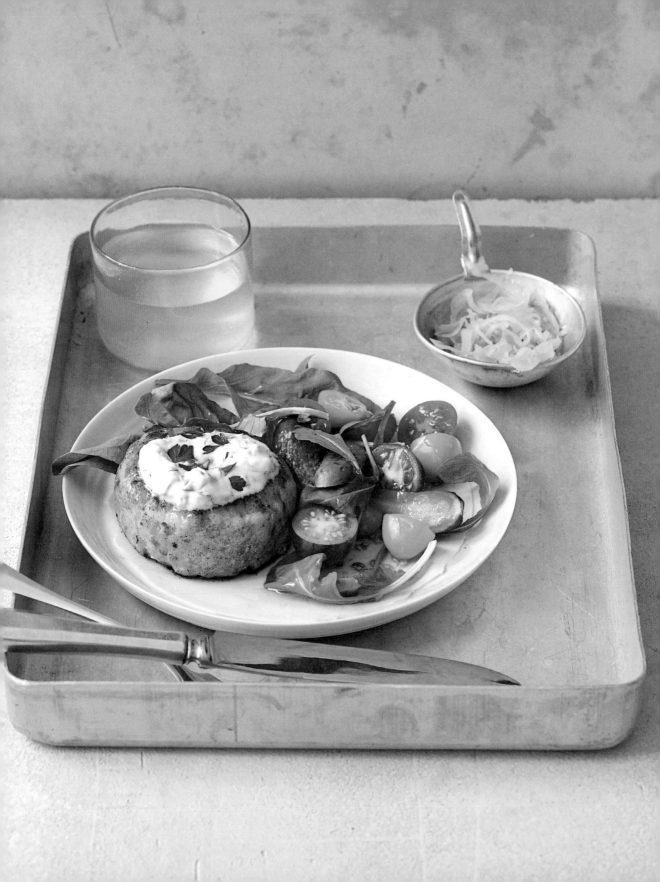

CAULIFLOWER RICE:
TWO VARIATIONS

I loved cauliflower rice before I ever made it because I knew it meant I could eat a giant bowl of what felt like carbs, but wasn't. Sign me up! Now, this is a weekly staple in my house. Here, I explain the basic technique and then provide two different flavour profiles so it works for any menu or type of dish. You can also make a super basic sautéed 'rice' in oil with onions and garlic without any of the additional ingredients.

MAKES 2–4 SERVINGS

MOROCCAN-STYLE:

1 head cauliflower

2 tablespoons extra-virgin olive oil

30g flaked almonds

1 onion, finely chopped

1 carrot, finely diced

½ teaspoon ground cinnamon

80–120ml vegetable or chicken stock, or

bone broth (see page 111)

50g sultanas (or raisins)

2 teaspoons orange zest

⅛ teaspoon cayenne pepper

2 tablespoons chopped fresh chives

ASIAN-STYLE:

1 head cauliflower

2 tablespoons untoasted sesame oil

50g cashew nuts, chopped

1 onion, finely chopped

30g broccoli, finely chopped

½ teaspoon finely chopped fresh ginger

80–120ml vegetable or chicken stock, or

bone broth (see page 111)

2 teaspoons lime zest

⅛ teaspoon chilli flakes

2 tablespoons chopped fresh Italian or

Thai basil

Directions for either variation:

1 Chop the cauliflower florets and some of the stems (I save the rest for snacking!) into small pieces and pulse them in a food processor until they are the consistency of rice. Do not over-chop.

2 In a large frying pan, heat the oil over low-medium heat and sauté the nuts until they are golden and become fragrant, about 2–3 minutes.

3 Add the onions, carrots (or broccoli), and cinnamon (or ginger) and stir well, cooking for 3 minutes.

4 Add the cauliflower rice from the food processor and cook for 1 minute.

5 Add 80ml stock, the raisins (if using), citrus zest and cayenne pepper (or flakes) and cook for another 10–15 minutes, or until you feel it is fully cooked and flavours are well-combined. Add more stock if needed to sauté. Taste and adjust seasoning if necessary.

6 Garnish with the fresh herbs and serve immediately.

CLASSIC CURRY

A delicious dish that warms your cells from the inside out, this customisable Indian-style curry is filling, healthy and a total party in your mouth. Below I've provided two options, vegetarian-style Sweet Potato and Rapini or Chicken and Chickpeas. I like to serve the curry over traditional basmati rice or quinoa, or just on it's own.

MAKES 2–4 SERVINGS

1 tablespoon melted coconut or extra-virgin olive oil

3 large garlic cloves, crushed or chopped

1 onion, sliced into half moons

1 carrot, finely diced

2 tablespoons curry powder

½ teaspoon ground cinnamon

½ teaspoon ground coriander

1 teaspoon ground turmeric

Sea salt and freshly ground black pepper

1 × 400ml can coconut milk, light or regular

240ml vegetable or chicken stock, or bone broth (see page 111)

1 × 400g can white beans, rinsed and drained

1 small bunch kale, any variety, de-stemmed and chopped

1 Heat the oil in a large non-stick pan over medium–high heat and sauté the garlic, onion and carrot for 7–8 minutes, until the carrot begins to soften.

2 Add the curry powder, cinnamon, coriander and turmeric; season with sea salt and pepper and mix to coat the vegetables. Cook for a further 2–3 minutes, allowing the spices to warm through and flavour the vegetables.

3 Pour the coconut milk and stock into the pan and mix thoroughly.

4 Add the white beans and kale; cover and continue to cook until the vegetables are soft and flavours are well combined, 5–7 minutes.

5 Taste and adjust the seasonings, adding more sea salt and pepper or more curry powder. Serve immediately.

SWEET POTATO AND RAPINI VARIATION

200g sweet potato or winter squash, chopped

Extra-virgin olive oil or coconut oil

Sea salt and freshly ground black pepper

350g rapini, or broccoli florets

Season the sweet potato with oil, salt and pepper. Roast at 190°C/gas mark 5 until caramelised, about 35–50 minutes. Add it and the rapini or broccoli florets to the curry mixture in Step 4 as a swap for the white beans and kale.

CHICKEN AND CHICKPEAS VARIATION

1 tablespoon coconut oil or ghee

140g salted boneless chicken (with or without skin depending on preference), chopped

1 × 400g can chickpeas, rinsed and drained

Sear the chicken in coconut oil or ghee until lightly browned. You can also swap with pre-cooked organic rotisserie chicken, shredded. Add it and the chickpeas to the curry mixture in Step 4 instead of white beans and kale.

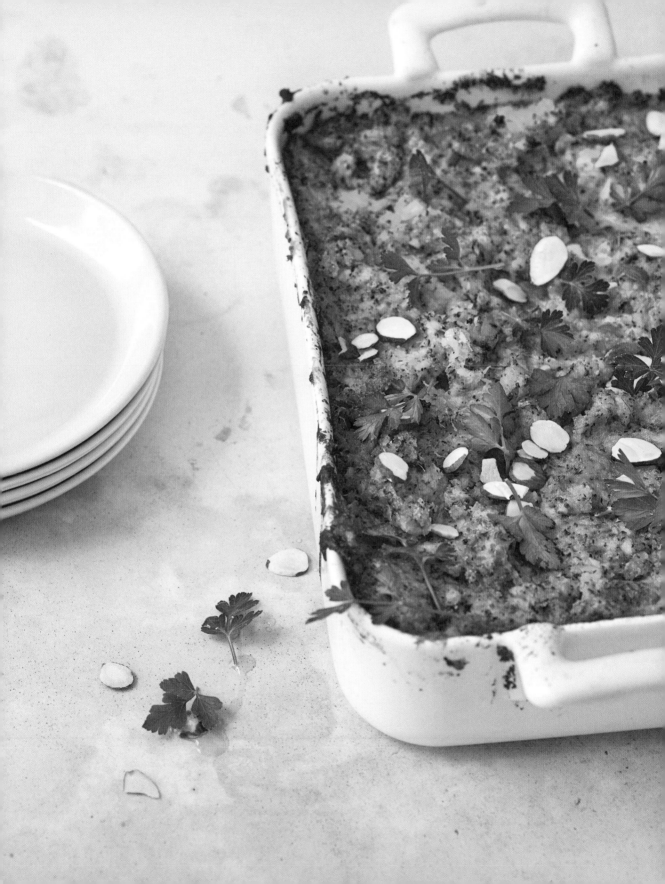

SHEPHERD'S PIE

Ideal for a bring-and-share supper, this pie satisfies everyone's tastebuds and makes great leftovers. I also love to make the mash on its own and pair it with a simple seared protein like salmon or tempeh for an easy weeknight meal.

MAKES 6–8 SERVINGS

1 recipe Happy Joes (see page 51)

SWEET POTATO AND BROCCOLI MASH

1 large sweet potato, chopped (or use regular sweet potato or yam)

1 large head broccoli, chopped (florets only, save stems for snacking)

½ teaspoon sea salt

1 tablespoon extra-virgin olive oil, butter or ghee

OPTIONAL GARNISHES:

Chopped fresh parsley and/or coriander

Toasted flaked almonds

Shredded red cabbage, raw or 'quick pickled' by soaking in 60–120ml cider vinegar (enough to just cover the cabbage) while pie is cooking

1 Preheat the oven to 190°C/gas mark 5.

2 Steam the sweet potato for 10 minutes.

3 Add the broccoli to the pan and steam for a further 10 minutes, until easily pierced with a fork or knife.

4 Transfer the broccoli and sweet potato to a food processor with the salt and oil or butter and pulse until combined (see Tip).

5 Line a 33 × 23cm baking dish with the Happy Joes mixture, then top it with a layer of the mash.

6 Bake until completely heated through and the mash starts to brown a bit, about 15–25 minutes. For a browned and crispy top, finish under the grill for a further 5–10 minutes. Serve with garnishes of choice.

tip

For a smooth mash consistency you'll want to stop the food processor after the sweet potato and broccoli are mostly combined and scrape down the sides with a spoon. Continue pulsing as directed.

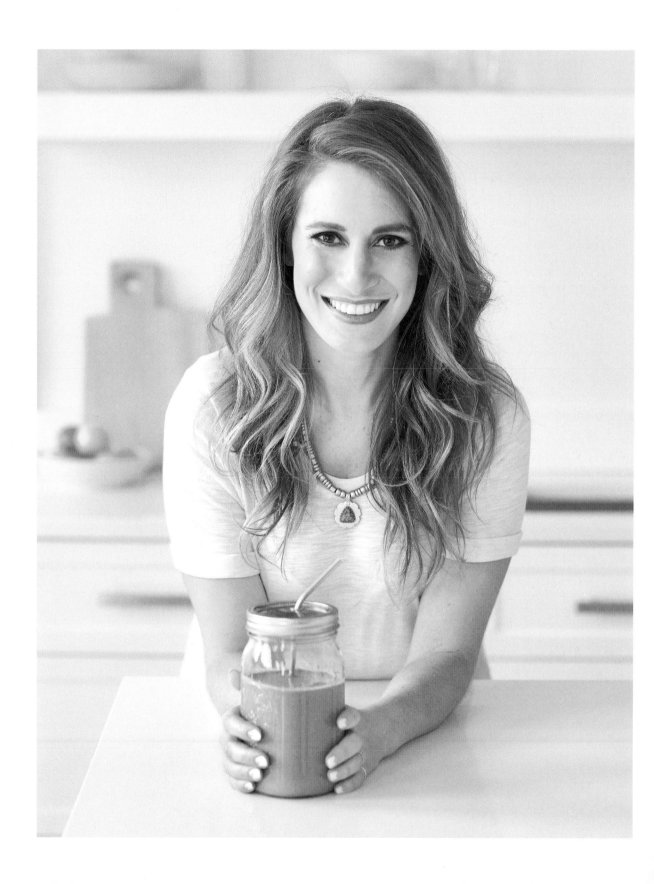

CHAPTER 4

DRINK

If your poop is the boat, how can it travel without a river?

We constantly obsess about food, but how much attention do we pay to what we drink? Our hydration habits have far-reaching consequences, affecting cell replenishment and appetite levels. If you hydrate in an 'upgraded' way from the top of your day, those energy dips and fierce appetite spikes are less likely to happen and will be less manic when they do.

It's a no-brainer that having a Double Caramel Venti Frappuccino with extra caramel and extra whip (not an exaggeration; I overheard someone ordering this next to me at a Starbuck's) at 3pm is not exactly good for your booty (inside or out). Similarly, drinking water laced with aspartame, high fructose corn syrup, or any of that other fancy junk is using a perfect delivery system – liquid – to flood your fine form with poison.

Getting your energy from sugar and caffeine relies on artificial stimulants instead of healthy ones. Here's the deal with coffee: it looks awesome in a porcelain mug on your Instagram when you're sitting in the café window on a beautiful street. Coffee is a ritual. It's warming on cold days and cooling on hot ones, and you can turn it into grown-up dessert to-go (or rely on it as an appetite suppressant, but no one really wants to admit that one). I am the first one to get excited about a beverage that gets all dressed up with dusted cinnamon. But here it is: coffee, in the way we commonly consume

it (overly processed and from poor-quality sources), is dehydrating, acidic and, depending on how and where it's grown, can be chock full of chemical pesticides. Additionally, coffee usually ends up as the perfect vehicle for completely unhealthy artificial sweeteners and chemical creamers.

But the biggest point I want to make about coffee is less about the beverage itself and more about the habits that typically go along with being a regular large latte drinker. Coffee's famous sidekick is a croissant/muffin/little yummy-snacky-cakey-sugary cookie thing or, worse, nothing at all. Starting your day with your morning coffee often equates to skipping breakfast and not taking care of yourself at the critical beginning of your day. Coffee becomes that saving grace from home to meeting, there to comfort you and provide the worst kind of 'sustenance'; that little life raft to get you through one part of your day and onto the next unhealthy choice; the auto-pilot crutch that keeps us from going inside and exploring what our belly, body or life is really asking for.

If you can't give up your morning cup of java without a monster, pounding headache or feeling too tired to think straight, it's a problem. You want to be able to wake feeling rested with sufficient energy to be alert and, even if you're not exactly a cheery morning person, to at least be a functional one without needing a stimulant. I'm not putting down all coffee drinkers. If you are able to drink coffee without dependency, be it your high-quality homemade 'butter' coffee

(blended with nourishing fats like butter and MCT or coconut oil, a.k.a., 'Bulletproof Coffee') or that delicious Americano at a healthy brunch, then you won't hear me trying to stop ya! Heck, I'll likely even join you. But do you see the difference?

UPGRADED HYDRATION

Rather than saying 'never', there is always an option to upgrade to a better choice or swap one habit for another that provides the same benefit without the downside. One of my common behaviour upgrades is when I choose to go to dance class or go for a quick run in the mornings. Exercising when I first wake up makes my morning pleasant; I start my day feeling rested with less stress and more natural energy.

So what do I mean by 'upgraded hydration'? First, the majority of the fluids you drink throughout the day need to be water. Yes, teas, coconut water and kombucha all count as liquids, but your body, of which 60 per cent is made of water, really needs the pure H2O. Water does it all. It helps form your saliva, regulates your body temperature through sweating, lubricates your membranes, joints and spinal cord and is vital to brain function. And when it comes to digestion, water is your river. A full, flowing river is essential to a healthy body and a balanced state of mind.

For optimal hydration, drink filtered water that eliminates impurities such as chlorine and heavy metals and is slightly alkaline. Your body's pH level, the measurement of acidity in your body, can have a massive impact on how you feel. Whereas a particular food or drink may be very acidic and good for you, the overall acidity levels in the body need to be balanced. While your stomach needs a higher level of acidity to break down food, your mouth should be more alkaline (think less acidic on the pH level scale). The meals you make from my recipes and the nutritional principles from this book will naturally lead to a healthy pH balance within the body. The foods that I ask you to reduce or eliminate – the sugars, processed carbs, factory-farmed meats – although not acidic outside the body are acid promoting to the extreme inside your body. The foods you will upgrade to – greens, healthy fats and seeds for example – are naturally alkaline. One of the easiest ways to alkalise your body first thing in the morning is to drink a giant jar of filtered

tip

Despite advertisements, your stomach needs a critical level of acid to properly digest your food and drink. When you take an antacid and artificially lower the acid levels in your stomach, your body eventually produces more to compensate. This can lead to a longer-term dependence on the drug to maintain proper acid balance.

THINK OF WATER AS A BLANK CANVAS ON WHICH YOU CAN CREATE ANY FLAVOUR TASTE YOU CRAVE

water with lemon or lime. Although lemons and limes are technically acidic, they contain minerals potassium, magnesium and sodium, which, when metabolised in your body, create a beautiful alkaline effect.

Water doesn't have to be boring. If you think of water as a blank canvas on which you can create any flavour or taste you crave, depending on your mood or needs, it becomes exciting. There are so many fun things you can add to water: a splash of aloe vera juice, fresh orange juice, a squeeze of lime, mint leaves, cucumber spears, sliced strawberries … You are the bartender.

A few notes on water:

★ Don't drink water with meals. It will dilute your gastric juices (especially your HCL, the acid in your stomach). Aim to finish a beverage 30 minutes before each meal and wait an hour after before drinking more.

★ Avoid adding ice to your water; it puts out your belly's 'fire'. (In Ayurvedic medicine, an ancient system of healing created by the sages in India over 5,000 years ago, digestion is called jatharagni – the 'internal fire', or your metabolic life force.)

★ Make sure you drink enough water each day.

Here is a good formula to calculate how much you need, so you don't have to think about it again. Simply divide your body weight in kilograms by 30 and this is the number of litres you want to drink each day. An average glass typically contains about 25 centilitres so you can easily determine how many glasses

you need. For example, a person who weighs 60kg will need to drink about 2 litres, or eight glasses of water a day. Almost everyone falls short of their daily requirement, so I created the following routine to help you increase your water consumption. Fill up a 500ml handled jar with filtered water and place it on your bedside table before you go to sleep. Then first thing in the morning drink it periodically while performing your morning routine, whether it's getting ready for work, exercise or breakfast. Before you head out the door you'll already have consumed a quarter of your eight glasses of water for the day! This should help you reach your desired water intake and create a happier, more naturally pH-balanced belly and body.

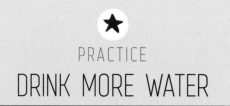

PRACTICE

DRINK MORE WATER

Purchase a quality water filter for your home.

Gather some large glass bottles or handled jars from a local car-boot sale or second-hand shop, or buy new ones or order them online.

Show me your bedside table jar with the hashtag #GoWithYourGutBook.

Start each day by drinking your big ol' beautiful jar of water before you leave the house (or get on to your morning to-do list).

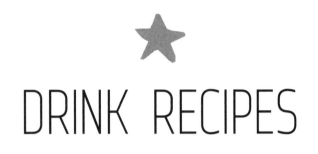

DRINK RECIPES

Let's get flowing! The following recipes will have you downright excited to nourish and hydrate that beautiful body of yours. When you are hydrated, your digestion and your life starts to flow easily. From sweet to savoury, I've got you covered for all sorts of occasions. Bottoms up!

Water Flavour Chart
Slim From Within Water
Short-cut Alternative Milk
Green Protein Smoothie
Cinnamon Toast Smoothie
Savoury Smoothie
Rose and Berry Smoothie
Green Juice
Best Bitters Soda

WATER FLAVOUR CHART

Need some H2O inspiration?
You can mix and match these ingredients to make your own fabulous water creation.

★

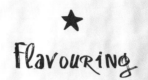

Basil | Coriander

Mint | Cinnamon sticks

Lavender | Ginger

Rosemary | Vanilla pod

★

Fruits and veggies

All berries	Pomegranate	Peaches
Grapefruit	Cucumber	Kiwi
Lemon	Watermelon	Apple
Orange	Cantaloupe	Pear
Lime	Honeydew	Tomato
Pineapple	Nectarines	Fennel

SLIM FROM WITHIN WATER

Here is a great way to de-bloat your body. This works during colder AND warmer months by combining natural diuretics and detoxifying ingredients into one delicious glass. Cucumber and lemon work to alkalise your body, while the cayenne and ginger jumpstart your metabolism and aid in flushing out your organs. Making a big jug of it this way also ensures that you'll be drinking lots of delicious and lightly flavoured water. Aim to have one jug every one or two days.

MAKES 2 LITRES

2 litres water

1 teaspoon freshly grated ginger

1 medium cucumber, peeled and thinly sliced

1 medium lemon, thinly sliced

Juice of 2 limes

½ teaspoon cayenne pepper

1 Combine all the ingredients in a large jug and stir!

2 Cover and refrigerate.

SHORT-CUT ALTERNATIVE MILK

Although convenient, packaged alternative milks often contain too many not-so-good-for-you ingredients (like carrageenan, in particular), so I created this dairy-free 'short-cut' milk so you can make it in five minutes flat. It's perfect as a base for the smoothies in this chapter.

MAKES ABOUT 1–1.5L

1 litre water

150g unsweetened desiccated coconut (fastest version), unsalted cashew nuts or unsalted almonds (See Note)

Pinch of sea salt

1 or 2 stoned dates (optional, if you prefer a sweeter version)

Add the ingredients to a blender and blend at high speed until it reaches a milk-like consistency. You can strain the pulp from the mixture through a piece of muslin, but I typically use it just as-is!

★
NOTE

Soak cashew nuts in water for 20 minutes to 1 hour, then drain. Soak almonds for at least 20 minutes (or even overnight) before draining and using in milk.

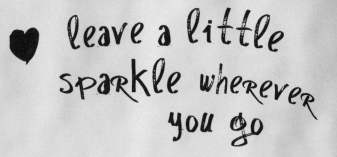

leave a little
sparkle wherever
you go

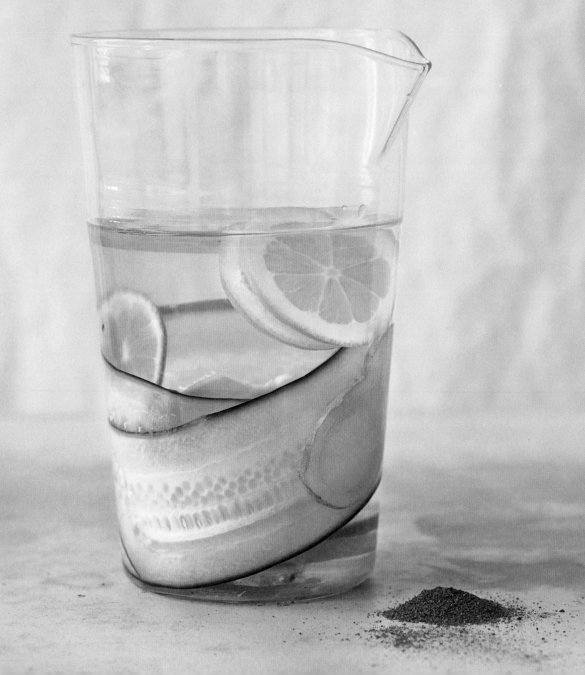

GREEN PROTEIN SMOOTHIE

I've come a long way since my first healthy recipe, the green smoothie, but I wanted to include it because it's simple, delicious and still a summertime staple for me. If you make this multiple times a week, don't forget to switch up your greens for maximum nutritional value. With the add-ins, remember to keep it simple: only one or two at a time works best. Feel free to play around with the ratios to see what you like best: more or less water for a thinner or thicker smoothie, for example.

MAKES 1 SERVING

1 scoop protein or 1 tablespoon
collagen powder

240ml homemade Alternative Milk (recipe on
page 72), coconut water or water

4 or 5 ice cubes

1 banana or 50g berries (frozen works best),
or anything that's in season

70g chopped kale or spinach (can use the
organic, pre-washed varieties)

1–2 tablespoons chia seeds

1 small piece of avocado (1 or 2 tablespoons
for creaminess and additional fat, optional)

OPTIONAL ADD-INS
(CHOOSE ONLY 1 OR 2 EACH TIME)

1 teaspoon ground cinnamon (or more;
cinnamon is great for your metabolism and
adds a lot of nice flavour)

1 tablespoon nut or seed butter

1–2 teaspoons ground flax meal (if you
have a powerful blender you can use the
whole seeds)

½ teaspoon spirulina

1 tablespoon raw cacao or carob powder

1–2 teaspoons maca powder

1 Add all the ingredients to a blender, along with one or two add-ins, if using. Blend on low. Once everything starts to combine, you can switch it to high and blend away. You may need to scrape the sides of the blender down with a spoon once or add an additional splash of liquid.

2 Taste and add more ice cubes if needed. Pour into a tall glass and enjoy!

CINNAMON TOAST SMOOTHIE

Sometimes you just want a bowl of Curiously Cinnamon. Or is that just me? So here it is, totally healthified and served up in a tall glass. Plus, cinnamon is high in antioxidants and acts as an anti-fungal, antibacterial and anti-inflammatory (which protects against heart disease). In addition, cinnamaldehyde, the compound responsible for most of the health benefits, has been shown to reduce insulin resistance and lower blood sugar levels, making it a powerful anti-diabetic!

MAKES 1 SERVING

120ml homemade Alternative Milk (recipe on page 72) or shop-bought alternative milk (cashew or coconut works best)

2 tablespoons protein or collagen powder

½ teaspoon ground cinnamon

4–6 ice cubes

1 frozen banana

½ teaspoon maca powder

1 Combine all the ingredients with 120ml water in a blender and blend on high speed.

2 Pour into a glass and sprinkle with additional cinnamon before serving.

SAVOURY SMOOTHIE

This savoury smoothie is my pride and joy. So many of my holistic friends are on the smoothie bandwagon but, as I explained, a cold smoothie first thing in the morning isn't always the best thing to get your digestive system going. Since smoothies are convenient and such a great way to get more nutrients in your bod, I set out to create one, utilising gut-friendly bone broth! Thus, the savoury smoothie was born. Somewhere between a smoothie and a soup, it's a perfect way to start your day or rev up your afternoon.

MAKES 1 SERVING

120ml bone broth (see recipe on page 111 or purchase from a quality source), cold or room temperature

1 cucumber, peeled and chopped

10g fresh coriander, chopped

Juice of 1 lemon

15g spinach leaves

2 celery sticks, chopped

Pinch of sea salt (optional)

1 Combine all the ingredients in a blender. Blend until totally smooth, but try to avoid over blending as this will create a lot of foam.

2 Add more bone broth, if needed, to reach the texture you want.

3 Pour into a glass or bowl and enjoy!

ROSE AND BERRY SMOOTHIE

My favourite ice cream in Los Angeles is from this classic Middle Eastern shop, Mashti Malone's. They serve up a flavour you rarely find – rose essence. Since I rarely eat traditional ice cream, I knew I had to recreate that delicious and sweet rose flavour in an everyday less dairy-intensive way. This smoothie is light, bright and a perfectly sweet treat. And a bonus: rose is wonderful for your digestive system. I like to think of rose essence as a superfood for your belly. It's known in the Ayurvedic world as soothing, cooling and moisturising, both inside and out.

MAKES 1 SERVING

240ml homemade Alternative Milk (recipe on page 72) or shop-bought alternative milk, vanilla or plain

50g berries, frozen or fresh

½ frozen banana

1 teaspoon pure rose essence

1 tablespoon collagen powder (optional)

Ice cubes (optional)

1 Combine all the ingredients in a blender and enjoy.

GREEN JUICE

Light and bright, this is my favourite green juice recipe, featuring three of my favourite ingredients to juice: grapefruit, a wonderful natural detoxifier; cucumber, hydrating for your body and nourishing for your skin; and mint. In addition to being great for digestion, mint makes this juice super delicious. I've also added a little healthy fat in the form of coconut oil or chia seeds to help your body absorb the nutrients from your freshly juiced produce.

MAKES 1–2 SERVINGS

½ grapefruit, peeled

1 cucumber

10g fresh mint leaves

70g chopped kale or spinach

2.5cm piece fresh ginger, peeled

1 lime, peeled

½–1 pear or green apple (optional)

½ teaspoon coconut oil or chia seeds

1 Using a juicer, juice all the ingredients except the oil or seeds.

2 Pour into a glass and add the oil or seeds and enjoy.

BEST BITTERS SODA

While I am not one for soda, I sometimes crave a little fizzy deliciousness, and my clients do too! That's why I created a homemade soda that incorporates great-for-your-gut digestive bitters. This drink is wonderful for settling the stomach.

MAKES 2–3 SERVINGS

Juice of ½ lemon

Juice of ½ orange

2–4 drops of herbal bitters

240ml sparkling water or water kefir

Ice

1 teaspoon fresh ginger juice (optional)

1 Mix all ingredients together in a large screw-top jar or small jug.

2 Serve immediately or refrigerate for up to one day.

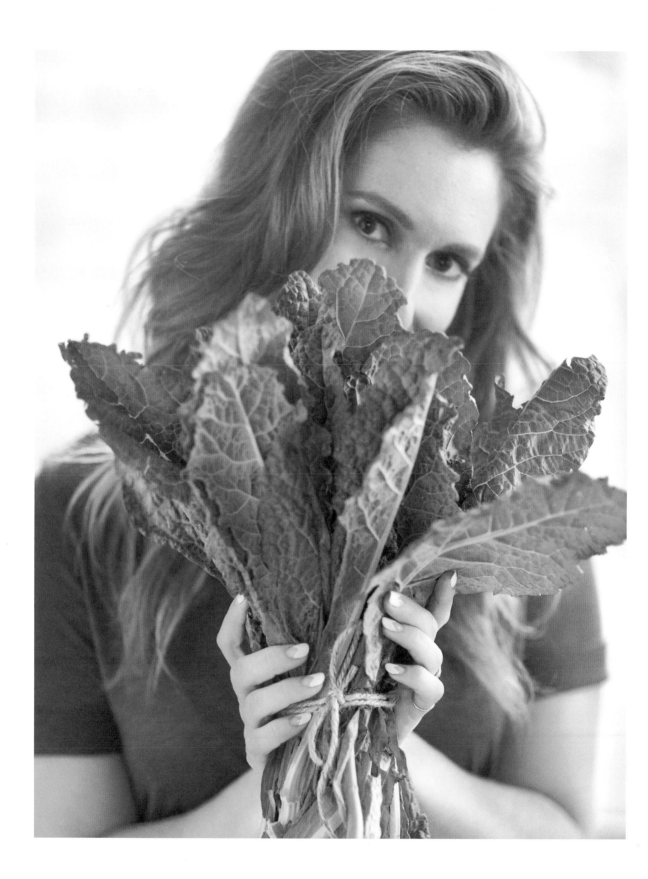

CHAPTER 5

FLOW

When in your life have you felt 'stopped up?' Chances are, when you take a moment to consider the question, you will realise that when you were blocked in your head or heart, you were blocked in the tail-end too. The inverse also holds true though, and this is something I am constantly teaching: movement inside creates movement in your life. The goal is to create a sense of flow that carries from our insides to our outsides, from our physical beings to how we experience our daily lives. None of these tummy functions are just about diet alone.

What does it mean to you to be 'blocked?' Just saying the word reminds me of a choking feeling; I think of being unable to express myself creatively or make a decision (a charming Libra quality of mine). I think 'trapped, stuck, backed-up or unable to take a leap of faith'. If you think back to a day or week when your bowels were not regular, how were you feeling in your career, in your relationships?

OK, now think of the word 'flow'; what is possible when you are flowing? What visualisations do you have? I imagine myself in ballet class as my arms swoop through the air. I am letting go of my inner critic, who is busy comparing me with the more advanced dancers, and I just move freely without inhibition. Or when my home feels calm and clean. Or that moment when I ask for something of the universe and all of a sudden, an email appears in my inbox that basically says, 'Here you go!' Our bowels, which can be flowing or blocked, are integral to our bodies

and our bodies are integral to our minds and every experience we have.

LET'S TALK ABOUT POOP

Pooping is your digestive system's job, as in top of the resumé. Are you someone who 'can't go' when you travel or until you've had your first cup of coffee? Does pooping stress you out? Telling yourself 'I just don't go' is like telling yourself you won't get the job before you've even had the interview. It isn't your body that is failing to work for you, it is your body that is speaking to you. It is telling you something is off and asking you for help.

OK friends, so do you want to know what technically happens when you're stopped up? According to the Johns Hopkins University Medical Library definition, constipation occurs when the colon absorbs too much water. Normally, as food moves through the colon (also known as your lovely large intestine), the colon absorbs water from the food while forming stool (waste products). Muscle contractions then push the stool towards the rectum and, by the time the stool reaches the rectum, most of the water has been absorbed, making the stool solid. When the colon's muscle contractions are slow or sluggish, which can occur due to stress, medication or a lack of water, fibre and physical activity, the stool moves through the colon too slowly, resulting in too much water absorption. As I mentioned earlier, water is literally your poop's life raft.

My pro-poop recipe! It consists of six things:

1 Breathing and slowing down
2 Water
3 Chewing
4 Diet: what we are putting into our mouth
5 Quieting our mind
6 Moving our body

Like all the connections I make between your mind and body, this one's another biggie: physical movement helps your organs move and function, too. This includes your digestion. Physical movement gets the blood pumping, the juices flowing, the energy going ... you follow what I'm saying?

When I run or walk outside, I think of it as moving myself forward, not just physically, but mentally. It's less about my body and more about my thoughts; it sparks my natural creativity. I feel like I am getting things done.

In terms of your digestion, just think: your organs are filled with living breathing microorganisms that need your love and attention. It's important to remember that these organs like to be moved. This little cellular family likes to be considered, brought into awareness, to be twisted and wrung out from the core. Stretched. Rolled. Whether that's through some yoga twists or self-massage, when you are lifting those limbs and doing something – anything – you are sparking what's going on inside, too.

Now that that we've made that important connection between the belly and the body as a whole, let's get into the topic that always comes up when it comes to being regular: fibre.

WHAT ABOUT FIBRE?

In my childhood house, bran muffins baked using the recipe on the side of the All-Bran box were a staple. I can't think of our kitchen without seeing a picture of my mother scooping the batter into her beloved 40-year-old muffin tins. One whiff of that bready, sweet scent has the power to take me back to those yummy, homey goodies. Not the worst possible scenario for establishing regularity, but as far as your bowels are concerned, fibre from wheat bran plus processed sugar is not the upgraded *Go With Your Gut* way to go. High-fibre cereals can help you go, but have you noticed they also give you excess gas and other discomforts? Not ideal.

tip

There are four qualities of a perfect poop:

1) how often you go (ideally 1–3 times a day)

2) the consistency of your stool (ideally soft and long the majority of the time)

3) how easy it is to pass, the length of time you spend in the bathroom (ideally 2–5 minutes)

4) you are able to get it all out

WHEN I RUN OUTSIDE, I THINK OF IT AS MOVING MYSELF FORWARD, NOT JUST PHYSICALLY, BUT MENTALLY.

A friend of mine told me that, although she is in her thirties, her mother still foists jumbo-sized containers of Metamucil on her when they get together. When she protests, her mother says, 'My doctor tells me to take it every day! He says it's good for your father!' One of my clients confessed that she has been using laxatives since she was 11 years old when she began buying the synthetic chocolate squares from the pharmacy. She suffered from haemorrhoids and, at the time she started working with me, could not produce a bowel movement without taking a pill. Here's the thing: highly processed, artificial and, in my client's case, potentially toxic products exacerbate the problem that an advertiser has convinced you it solves. If you really want to start going for number twos with soothing, dependable, easy, comfy, cosy regularity, there are some things that you need to understand about fibre, about how it works in your body and about how to get more of the right kinds of it.

Please remember that with all dietary changes, I want you to start small and work your way up.

The less dramatic you make this, the easier it is to continue doing. If you go from eating tons of junk food to buckets of kale and cabbage, you are going to experience a lot of gassiness. The kind of fibre, a.k.a. roughage, that you want to be eating is of the plant and wholegrain variety, coming from vegetables, fruits, beans, nuts, seeds or wholegrains. Nature delivers us this whole and perfect fibre package; there is no need to go the artificial route.

Dietary fibres are the parts of the plant foods that are undigested by your body and that pass through the stomach, small intestine, colon and out of your body, absorbing water along the way and facilitating bowel movements. The two kinds of dietary fibre are soluble and insoluble. The National Institute of Health's U.S. National Library of Medicine website gives a good definition of soluble and insoluble fibres: Soluble fibre attracts water and turns to gel, slowing down the digestion. Soluble fibre is found in oat bran, barley, nuts, seeds, beans, lentils, peas and many fruits and vegetables.

Insoluble fibre adds bulk to the stool and helps it pass through the body.

Some sources of insoluble fibre are wheat bran, seeds, nuts, barley, brown rice, bulgur, tons of root vegetables and their skins, courgettes, celery, broccoli, cabbage, onions, tomatoes, carrots, cucumbers, green beans, dark leafies and most fruits.

When shifting from a diet that lacks fibre, or one where you're just not getting enough of the right kinds, gradually lose the foods that sabotage the gut's ability to process and eliminate what you serve it. Little daily choice by little daily choice, replace them with better alternatives. You're having a meal anyway, so why not make it one that makes you feel physically and mentally great?

HELPFUL MOVE-YOUR-BOOTY GUIDELINES

1 Schedule your workouts or movement practice in advance. I have been going to some of the same classes every day for years now. They're blocked off in my calendar, I don't see clients then, and I say no to anything and everything that would interfere with that time. In response, the Universe does its part and never gives me anything at that time that I would have to miss! (and yes, the Universe will respond to your energy when you say something is unmovable and important). I recommend selecting a few workouts or classes each week and blocking them all out in your calendar now, for months, or at least at the start of each week. Then when your 7pm hip-hop reminder pops up on your phone, you'll be much more likely to go because your drinks with girlfriends didn't also get booked for that slot (it got booked for later because you told them you have a date with hip-hop before). See?

2 Get cute workout clothes you love (and I mean love). Being excited to spend time in your workout clothing can sometimes mean all the difference between getting to the gym or getting to your couch. It's fun to hang out in something you feel great in. One reminder though: don't wait until you have that 'perfect body' before investing in those clothes. No more 'when I have this, I'll get that'. You should live your life exactly the way you want it to be right now. No exceptions.

3 Try some of the fancy classes; they're worth it. If your city offers unique dance classes, fun spinning studios or anything else that sparks your interest, do them! I know they can be pricey, but they're often your best bet to actually enjoying your workout and being the most efficient with your time. These speciality classes and gyms create a sense of community and, deep down, we all really want to belong to something.

4 Explore the wonderful world of online workouts. The online workout community is incredible. There are so many inspiring teachers on YouTube or membership-type services so you'll never get bored! Many of them are free or offer a low subscription fee. You can check out some of my favourites at www. robynyoukilis.com/gutbookbonuses.

Part of the challenge in making the healthier choice is how available and attractive the wrong choices are in the store. You walk in and are immediately greeted by the rows of eye-popping colours. It's distracting. It's convenient. It's what you know. However, fresh produce comes in vibrant colours, too, and it's alive. And there are just as many options, just as much variety, in greens and veggies as in junk food – enough for a million whole and tasty meals. It's just about changing where you look in the store.

Maybe you love your cereal and think it does the trick. Or you love your fat-free, sugar-free bran muffin from the guy at the charming bakery you go to every Monday morning. The guy behind the counter loves you, too. He says 'Good morning!' and he has your muffin all ready for you before you can open your mouth to say 'Hello'. I just want to be really clear about this: I am not asking you to sacrifice foods you enjoy, just find better alternatives. I fully believe that the foods you can upgrade to are every bit as delicious, only they will agree with your body more.

My 'Good Poop List' (page 86) and the recipes that include these ingredients are no fail. If you eat more of these foods at each meal and less of the sugar-filled varieties that brag about their fibre content, you will be going more frequently. It's not that we don't know when something disagrees with us – our bodies show us in so many different ways – but how do we get from the awareness to acting on a different choice? Gradually begin to focus on the foods that have the flavour and power to do you good.

tip

One unusual item you'll always find in my bathroom is a Squatty Potty. This helpful device allows your body to sit in its natural position for relieving your bowels. You can check out some resources at www.robynyoukilis.com/gutbookbonuses.

CREATE YOUR CALM

Last, but not least, let's bring it back around to that mind/body connection. I want you to make this connection over and over again. Just like the limited amount of time we give ourselves to chew, we often give ourselves very little time in the loo! In earlier chapters, I asked you to slow down and allow yourself time to breathe and relax around your food. I asked you to turn off distractions and, if in a restaurant full of bustling activity or at the family dinner table on a stressful night, allow yourself to be centred and calm. No matter where you are and what emotions are in the room with you, you control your own energy and this, in turn, affects how your body processes what you feed it. You can create your own calm.

When you're in the bathroom, don't rush yourself! Allow yourself to go in there to breathe, relax, and take care of your business with ease. What is the bathroom like in your home? Is it painted in a soothing colour and uncluttered? How about the toilets in your workplace? Can you make these spaces feel more relaxing? Even joyful? The process of getting in touch with yourself will carry over to that public (or private) porcelain throne. Relax, zen-out, don't hurry. When you give your body time to rest and process without overload, it will thank you.

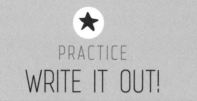

WRITE IT OUT!

At some point during my coaching process with clients, I assign them this exercise. We all have a poop story, but if you're like most of my clients (or most people in general), it could use a dramatic shift. Here's how:

Take out three individual pieces of paper and a pen. On the first one, write out everything you remember about what it was like for you to go for a number two as a baby or child. What does your mum tell you that you were like as a little one? How about the elementary school years? Were you like me and mistakenly thought you had a stomach ache every time you had to go? Any specific stories coming up for you? Write it all down.

Next, on the second piece of paper, write down anything and everything that's coming up for you as your current poop story. Can you go only at home now? How about when you travel? What's your home bathroom or office situation like? Does the very thought of hashing this out make you feel uncomfortable? Get it all down here.

And lastly, on a fresh new piece of paper, write out your 'new and empowering' story. Paint the scenario of what it will look and feel like for you to be someone who 'goes easily'. Include as many specifics and scenarios as you like. It will all help enrich this new picture and the new you you're stepping into.

GOOD POOP LIST

FERMENTED FOODS

Aim for local and organic, and they should always be unpasteurised and refrigerated. You want a living, growing product, so it is important to choose products that do not contain vinegar. Vinegar kills the live bacteria.

Favourites: Sauerkraut, kimchi, pickled vegetables, tempeh (fermented soybean cake), miso, kombucha (a fermented tea beverage – drink in much smaller portions than the bottle says; only up to 100ml at a time), beet kvass (another fermented beverage primarily made from beetroot and water)
Dairy based (if you can digest dairy): kefir, yogurts and cheeses, buttermilk
Unusual and fun: dosa, bean curd, natto, fermented breads such as sourdough and injera, fermented drinks such as amazake (Japanese rice drink), ginger beer, coconut water kefir (from fermented water kefir grains)

PREBIOTIC FOODS

Foods rich in prebiotics provide probiotics for the good bacteria in your gut. Think of them like food for the seeds you plant in your internal garden. Note that most of these foods must be eaten raw or lightly cooked to obtain the good gut benefits.

Favourites: dandelion greens and root, garlic, onions, leeks, green onions (anything from the allium family), Jerusalem artichokes, asparagus, bananas, plantains, honey, chicory (used in coffee substitutes), oats, jicama, apples

HEALTHY OILS AND FATS

All oils should be organic, cold-pressed and unrefined (you want them minimally processed and tampered with). Keep shelf-stable oils in a dark cupboard and away from sunlight so they don't oxidise. Any of the flavouring and medicinal oils benefit from being refrigerated.

Multi-use shelf-stable favourites: olive, coconut, red palm (sustainably sourced and harvested only), butter and ghee
Flavouring only (not to be heated): pumpkin seed, walnut, sesame, sacha inchi (a nut oil from the sacha inchi seed), avocado
Medicinal purposes: cod liver, evening primrose, flax

NUTS AND SEEDS

Always purchase organic, sprouted when possible and raw (or sprout them yourself by soaking in water, then drying). Nuts that have been commercially roasted, salted, etc. will add more salt and fat than you want and typically use poor-quality oils and salt. They can trigger other cravings as well. For example, I have a client who upgraded from overconsumption of sugar to overconsumption of tamari almonds. While the latter is technically a little better for her body and digestive system, it sabotaged her progress towards a healthier weight until we discovered this issue.

A note on flax seeds: whole flax seeds cannot be broken down and will pass through your digestive system unutilised. Grind fresh whole seeds in small batches with a spice grinder, or simply purchase as flax meal (but only if it's a heavily trafficked store and/or kept in the refrigerator aisle). Be sure to refrigerate them and use shortly after grinding.

Favourites: almonds, brazil, peanuts, macadamia, hazelnuts, pecans, cashews, walnuts, sunflower, sesame (I especially love a traditional macrobiotic seasoning called

gomasio – ground sesame seeds and sea salt), pumpkin, flax, chia, psyllium

Note: nuts are not popcorn! Mother Nature designed a nut perfectly – with a shell that's hard to crack so we would consume only a small serving at a time. This is a gentle reminde,r once again, that overconsumption of anything is tasking your belly with more than it needs and can deal with. In this case, with too much of a good thing – those healthy fats – so eat your nuts and seeds sparingly.

HEALTHY FAT-CONTAINING FOODS

Our bodies need fat to help us feel full and metabolise the nutrients we receive from the foods we eat. You want to make sure every meal you eat has some source of quality healthy fat from natural sources from this list or the Healthy Oils and Fats or Nuts and Seeds sections.

Favourites: Olives, coconut, avocado
Wild-caught oily fish: salmon, tuna, mackerel, herring, trout, sardines and anchovies.
Note: do not be afraid of eating the skin and little bones in your fish; they nourish your skin and bones, too

BONE BROTH

The collagen that breaks down from the connective tissue of bones simmered to make broth is an important component to help heal the lining of the gut. This creates a happier home for healthy bacteria. The bio-available minerals from the bones help increase mineral reserves in the body, making it more alkaline and supporting your body's natural buffering system.

Varieties: chicken, beef, turkey, fish, seaweed

GREENS AND HERBS

These provide perfect roughage for your colon. You'll want to aim to have an item from this list at every meal.

Favourites: kale (all varieties), dandelion, broccoli, rocket, collard greens, turnip greens, beet greens, spinach, mustard greens, all lettuces (romaine, radicchio, red or green leaf, frisée, mesclun), cabbage, Swiss chard, chicory, parsley, watercress, bok choy, fennel, dill, mint and more

DIGESTIVE-ENHANCING AND IMMUNE-BOOSTING FOODS

Favourites: turmeric, cardamom, coriander, cinnamon, cumin, caraway, ginger, cayenne pepper, black pepper, all peppers, garlic, lemon, onion
Bitters – from the health food store, not the kind used to make cocktails. You want them to be really bitter to produce digestive juices. Have a few drops before any meal

SUPPLEMENTS

Favourites: Aloe vera: soothing, cooling and calming; promotes growth of cells
Magnesium powder
Marshmallow root, licorice root, slippery elm bark: create a mucilaginous coating of the gut walls
Activated charcoal: eases digestion and removes toxins
Triphala: an Ayurvedic treatment
Spirulina and chlorophyll
Rose essence
Colostrum
Digestive enzymes
Immunity supplements such as olive leaf extract, echinacea and oil of oregano are great immune boosters and illness fighters

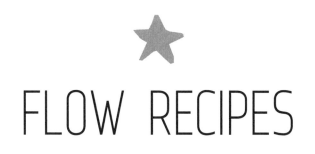

FLOW RECIPES

If I had my way, this greens and veggies section would've been the entire book. To get your flow going, you've got to get your roughage consumption up! I eat so many vegetables I should probably upgrade to a commercial-sized fridge. Here are my favourite recipes of all time. With these recipes, it has been a pure pleasure to turn veggie sceptics into believers.

Garlicky Restaurant-style Greens
Greens with Sweet Vinegar and Dried Fruit
Classic Roasted Root Veggies
Steamed Veggies
Curry- and Turmeric-Roasted Squash

GARLICKY RESTAURANT-STYLE GREENS

Ever wonder what restaurants do to make their kale, collard greens and spinach so yummy and why you can't ever make it taste the same at home? This recipe cracks the code on what restaurants do oh-so-well with their greens – they use tons of olive oil and garlic!

MAKES 2 SERVINGS

2–3 tablespoons extra-virgin olive oil
(2 for a smaller bunch of greens, 3 for larger sized greens)
1 bunch dark leafy greens, washed, stemmed, chopped and dried
2 or 3 garlic cloves, finely chopped or grated
(2 for a smaller bunch of greens, 3 for larger sized greens)
Sea salt and freshly ground black pepper
Squeeze of lemon juice (optional)

1 Heat 1–2 tablespoons of the oil in a large sauté pan over medium–low heat.

2 Add the greens and garlic, season generously with sea salt and pepper and mix well.

3 Sauté for 5–8 minutes, until the greens are soft and darken in colour.

4 Drizzle an additional tablespoon of olive oil over the greens and stir through. Scoop the greens from the pan and serve with a squeeze of lemon juice, if using.

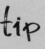

tip

Don't throw the stems away! You can chop them finely and add them to any recipe before the leafy parts of the vegetable, as they'll need a couple more minutes to cook than the more tender leaves. They also make great chewing toys for your dog!

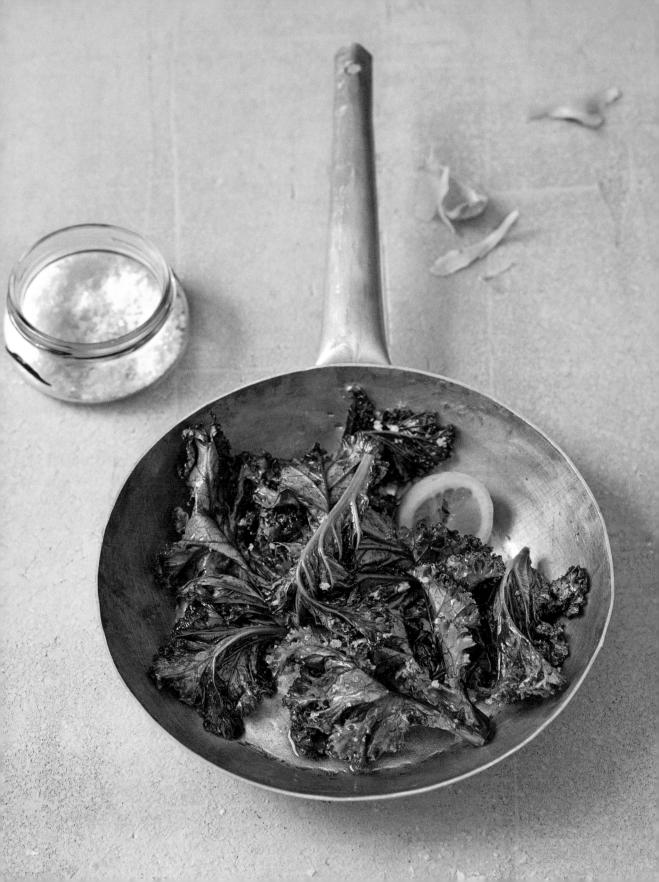

GREENS WITH SWEET VINEGAR AND DRIED FRUIT

This elevated version of sautéed greens is my go-to when I've been having too much of the usual garlic/lemon combo. The vinegar adds a tangy, bright and unusual flavour. Plus, anything with nuts and dried fruit always tastes extra delectable.

MAKES 2–3 SERVINGS

2 tablespoons raw nuts (pine, chopped cashews or cashew pieces and flaked almonds all work great)

1–2 tablespoons extra-virgin olive oil or coconut oil

3 garlic cloves, finely chopped or crushed

300g collard greens, mustard greens, kale or bok choy (be sure to de-stem if using collards, mustards or kale), chopped

Sea salt and freshly ground black pepper

3 tablespoons raisins, gogi berries, chopped prunes or currants

2 tablespoons balsamic or raw apple cider vinegar

1 Toast the nuts over medium heat in a dry frying pan for about 5 minutes, or until golden. Shake the pan often to keep the nuts from burning. Transfer them to a plate or bowl and set aside.

2 Heat the oil and garlic in a large frying pan, and sauté over medium heat for 1 minute, or until the garlic is fragrant.

3 Add the greens and season generously with salt and pepper. Stir, then cover the pan and cook for a further 2 minutes.

4 Add the dried fruit and nuts and stir. Cover and cook for 2 minutes.

5 Stir in the vinegar, cover and continue to cook for a further 1–2 minutes, until the greens are cooked through but not limp. Serve immediately.

tip

I'll typically use cashew pieces and flaked almonds in my recipes as they're already 'chopped' for you and eliminate an extra prep step. Plus they're usually less expensive and go further in recipes (because they have more volume) than whole nuts you chop or slice yourself.

CLASSIC ROASTED VEGGIES

Simple. Delicious. Straightforward. Vegetables really shine when perfectly roasted, allowing their natural sweetness to come through. Great for dinner the night you cook them (and borderline impossible to stop eating straight from the pan!), they're wonderful to have on hand throughout the week to spruce up salads and snack times.

MAKES 2–3 SERVINGS

300–400g chopped or sliced vegetable of choice, such as Jerusalem artichokes, leeks or onions

2 tablespoons oil of choice, such as coconut or sustainably produced and harvested red palm fruit

Sea salt and freshly ground black pepper

Fresh and dried herb of choice such as thyme or rosemary (optional)

1 Preheat the oven to 200°C/gas mark 6.

2 Spread the vegetables in a roasting dish. You'll want there to be a little space in between the veggies. Use an additional dish if necessary.

3 Toss them with the oil, a sprinkle of sea salt and the herbs. Roast for 20 minutes. Then check the veggies and turn the pan in the oven; keep cooking until the vegetables are fork tender and golden to dark brown all around. Taste and season them with additional salt and pepper, if needed.

VARIATIONS

Roasted Roots with Avocado: Roasted root veggies such as carrots, parsnips, beetroot, turnips or swede. After the veggies are cooked, serve with cubed avocado and the juice of 1 lemon.

Roasted Trees with Lemon and Chili: Roasted veggies such as cauliflower, romanesco or broccoli. After the veggies are cooked, serve with the juice and zest of 1 lemon, a small handful of chopped parsley and 1 teaspoon crushed chilli flakes.

Lime and Coriander Finished: Roasted veggies such as sweet potatoes or butternut squash. After the veggies are cooked, serve with the juice of 2 limes and a small handful of chopped fresh coriander..

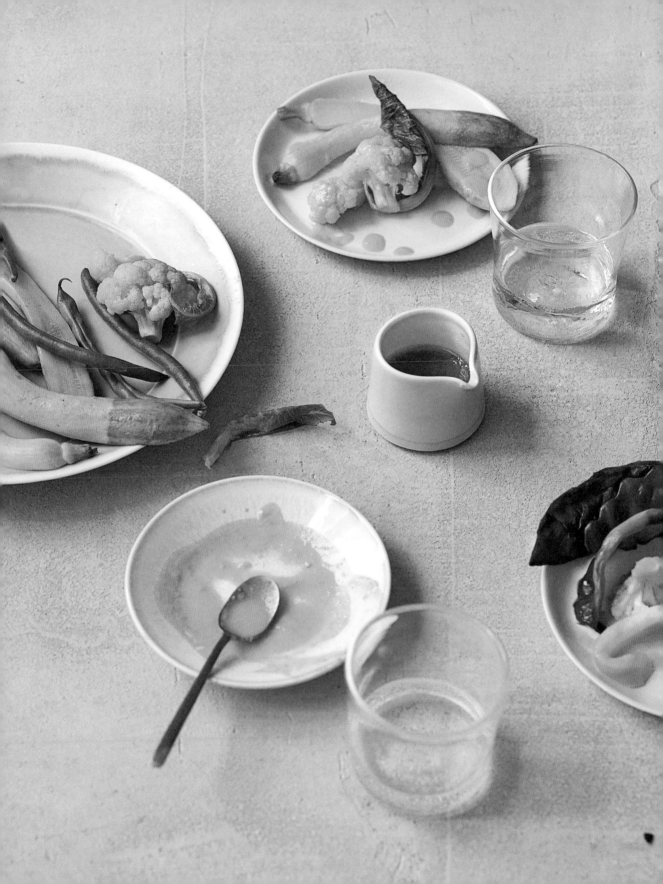

STEAMED VEGGIES

Considered the least 'cool' of all the cooking methods, steaming is one of the fastest, easiest and healthiest cooking methods out there. Fact: You can steam pretty much anything! Plus there's no sautéeing or measuring, so it's virtually foolproof. Just be sure to add enough water to the pan so you don't burn the bottom! Not like I've never done that before!

SERVING SIZE BASED ON AMOUNT OF VEGETABLES USED

Chopped or sliced vegetables of your choice

OPTIONAL INGREDIENTS:

Juice of ½ lemon

Extra-virgin olive oil or coconut oil

Sea salt and freshly ground black pepper

Fresh herbs

1 Fill a large pan with about 5cm of water and then fit it with a steamer basket. Put it over high heat and cover. Bring the water to a boil.

2 Once there's steam coming out of the pan, add your veggies and cover with a lid. (see Note).

3 Remove the veggies once they're fork tender or cooked to your liking. (Approximately 3–5 minutes for lighter, leafy vegetables and 7–10 minutes for denser and harder vegetables.) Serve them with a sauce or dressing or a simple squeeze of lemon juice, drizzle of olive oil and sprinkle of salt and pepper.

★
NOTE

Harder veggies will take longer to cook, while light leafy style veggies will cook quickly. I typically layer from longest cooking to shortest cooking times in the basket and then pull out veggies with tongs as they're ready!

tip

Don't have a steamer basket (yet)? You can do a variation on steamed vegetables by using a 'water sauté' method. Simply add 60–120ml of water to a large sauté pan over a high heat and cover. Once the pan is filled with steam, lower the heat to medium and cook until the vegetables are fork tender. Drain any excess water before serving.

CURRY- AND TURMERIC- ROASTED SQUASH

I visited my good friend Tricia in Newport Beach once and she made me kabocha squash prepared this way. Upon returning home, I think I made it every week for about three months straight! I couldn't stop craving, cooking and chatting about it! So nourishing for your body and satisfying for your bellies are they, you'll want to make these dense winter squashes a part of your weekly cooking routine.

SERVING SIZE BASED ON AMOUNT OF VEGETABLES USED

1 winter squash of choice (delicata, kabocha, butternut, hubbard, etc.), cubed or thinly sliced (Note: when buying organic, I'll generally cook and eat the peel too!)

2–3 tablespoons coconut oil

2 tablespoons curry powder

2 teaspoons ground turmeric

Sea salt

Freshly ground black pepper

1 Preheat the oven to 200°C/gas mark 6.

2 Spread the squash in a roasting dish. You'll want there to be space in between the pieces. Rub the squash with the oil.

3 Sprinkle it with the curry powder, turmeric and some sea salt.

4 Roast for 30–40 minutes, depending on thickness of the squash. The squash should be a rich golden yellow colour and browned a bit.

5 Taste and add some black pepper or more salt if needed. Serve immediately.

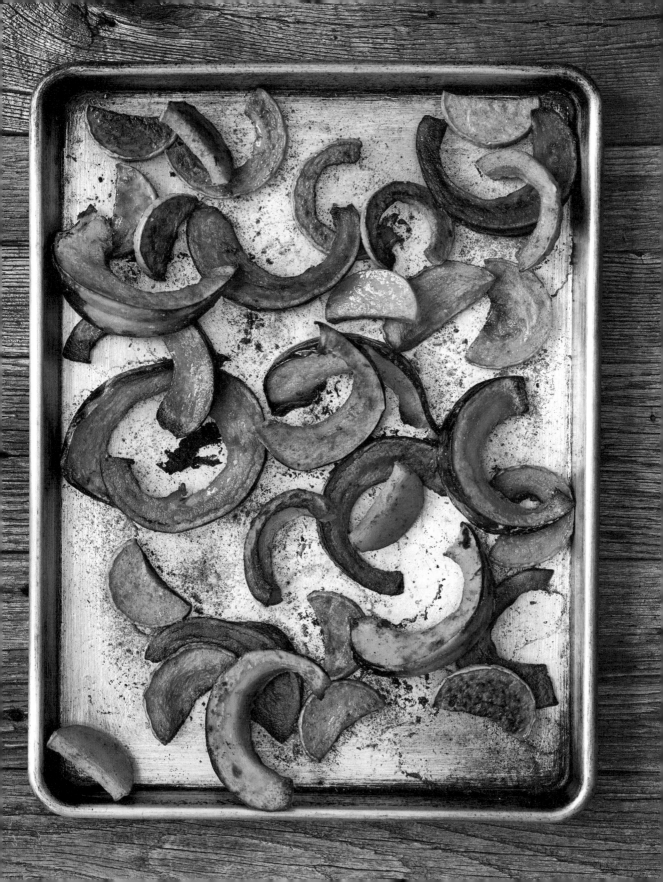

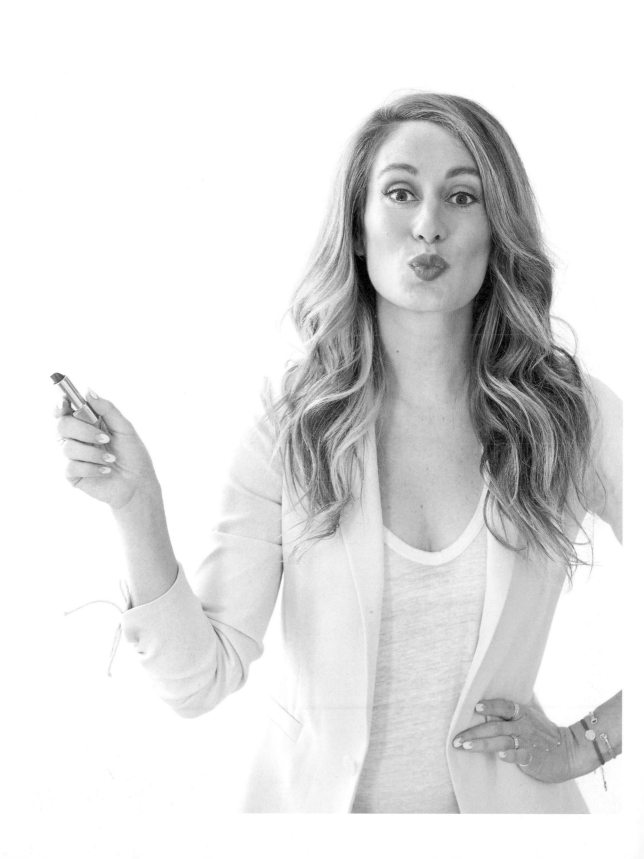

SHED

I can't tell you how often I hear during my group coaching calls, my ladies pleading to me about these two issues: belly bloat and what I call 'weight loss resistance', which is when they're doing everything 'right', but still not seeing a difference. It causes so much drama, anger and frustration that as we start our conversation, I am used to hearing a voice on the other end in a state of total emergency. When I designed one of my coaching programmes, I actually named one of the weekly lessons 'Why Is My Belly So Big?'. This is clearly an issue we are all dealing with in some form or another.

There are mental and physical elements to both weight-loss resistance and constantly feeling bloated. Everything that you practise in taking care of your digestive system will put you in a position to rationally approach how you feel about your body. By now you know there are many baby steps you can take to feel empowered about this, and it is not about the bloat or weight itself; it's about the entire range of habits that you are building.

IS IT ALL IN YOUR HEAD?

When we notice bloating, we usually notice the result of more than one factor, including our weight and, often, the size and shape of our belly. When it comes to carrying a higher percentage of fat on our bodies than we would like, I have never ever known it to be a strictly physical thing; there's always more there. So, yes, this book is about digestion and connecting to your gut, but it's also for my real girls. The ladies who know the complex connection between our physical and emotional selves, but can't seem to make the shifts stick.

So many of my one-on-one sessions have begun from the point of exhaustion when a client says, 'Robyn, I just want to be done with this'. Or, 'I thought I knew better'. Or, 'I thought I was done'. My response is always going to be, 'You may never be done with this', because that's the truth. Feeling fat is typically the result of noise in your head and less about what's happening on your hips. It's the feeling that's telling you what you're doing is wrong or is going to make you fat. Those thoughts might be happening every few days, or every few minutes. Our minds tend to be very busy places. In every moment, we have the power to see what is great or what is wrong with our bodies, what you love or what you want to fix.

Our busy minds are a part of our bodies and this relationship is lifelong, so wouldn't it feel nicer to speak to ourselves with some sweetness? Imagine your favourite little one, maybe a nephew or your best friend's child. Would you say any of the mean-spirited remarks we so carelessly aim at ourselves to them? Would you tell your favourite 4 year old, 'You have no business wearing that dress!' No, you wouldn't. And I don't want you speaking like that to yourself either (even when it's part of a well-timed joke).

In all my work, I still have moments (i.e. when trying on shorts) when I give my body a hard

time. Most of the time it's a harmless joke, but all the little comments add up. I'm a true New Yorker at heart – no matter how many times I wave the positivity wand I'll likely prefer the sarcastic and slightly snarky.

SO WHAT TO DO?

Go on a strict cleanse.

Not a juice cleanse, but a 'no-body-bashing' cleanse. Let's create a zero-tolerance rule around harmful and mean thoughts about our bodies. No more 'my butt makes a nice pillow' or 'my legs are strong, that's why they're on the bigger side'. These comments may sound 'cute' but secretly, they're mean.

Utilising the 'cleanse', we'll try to slowly reduce these types of negative thoughts to once a week, and then once a fortnight and then once a month. We'll create some space in between those moments, so when that feeling does come up, it doesn't affect you as dramatically, and you can recover faster. While you'll notice a significant change in just a few weeks, be patient in allowing these new habits to take hold. If you stick with it, these new thought muscles will get stronger and stronger, and so will your beautiful body.

THE BLOATING BREAKDOWN

Let's break down bloating so we can understand what's physically going on in that body of yours. Bloating is the distention of the abdomen, typically from gas produced by undigested food. Understanding this symptom is a little complicated, as it can happen for so many reasons – from eating too much and too fast to drinking too many fizzy drinks or chewing gum. Hormones and your menstrual cycle, as well as undiagnosed food intolerances, can also cause bloating. When a client comes to me complaining of constantly feeling bloated, I look at her diet. Is there a lot of sugar? Poor-quality salts? Gluten? Processed foods? Dairy? Even too many seemingly healthy foods at once? All of these can be causes of extra weight and feeling like a beached whale after every meal.

This bloating is also connected to the body's natural reaction to 'injury' or, in this case, a food you can't digest properly. Inflammation of this kind creates a double whammy against your energy supply. Your immune response gets activated, showing up as anything from bloating to hives to headaches, and your body has to spend a disproportionate amount of time and effort on digestion. This could be why you are so exhausted after eating particular foods. Chronic inflammation not only locks your fat cells in place and makes it hard to lose weight but also tends to accelerate diseases we might encounter later on in our lives, like heart disease, cancer and Alzheimer's.

THE TRUTH IS, TOO MUCH OF A GOOD THING IS STILL TOO MUCH.

The good news is you can fight this kind of inflammation by figuring out which foods your body might have allergies or intolerances to, and simplifying your meals with my 'Rule of 5'.

Identifying your food sensitivities will help you break through the wall of 'weight-loss resistance'. I recommend a simple elimination diet with the following steps: First, eliminate a food for 23 days. I'll typically start my clients with the most common culprits for digestive issues, such as gluten and dairy, but if you have an instinct to eliminate another food that might be causing you problems, go for it. On the 24th day, re-introduce one of the eliminated foods for two days in a row and see if you have any reaction whatsoever. Sensitivities or intolerances can show up as full reactions like hives, headaches or extreme bloating. They can also be on the subtler side like 'brain-fog' or just feeling 'off'. Remove the food once more on the third day and again see if you notice a difference. Then repeat with the other eliminated foods. If you feel better after isolating and removing the food both times (the 23 days AND the third day) it's a sign that this food or food type does not agree with your belly. You can also do additional rounds of eliminating soy, shellfish, alcohol,

peanuts and corn, all foods that commonly cause digestive issues. This information will empower you to finally know what to enjoy, and what to keep off your plate.

The easiest way to unburden your digestive system and get the most out of mealtime is to simplify your foods. I call this the Rule of 5: Eat no more than five different foods at any given meal. This is a gentle guide I created for my frustrated women who need to uncomplicate their plates and the overwhelming food 'noise' around them. Also, if you stick to the Rule of 5, you'll be more likely to say 'no thank you' when the crappy cookies come around! Preparation and finishing ingredients such as oil, herbs and spices do not count as part of the five.

The truth is, too much of a good thing is still too much. Whenever I pass by a popular freshly prepared salads to-go place at lunchtime, with its massive line out the door, I always think how hard a time all those bellies are going to have digesting those big 'ol plastic bowls of 25 supposedly 'healthy' salad toppings. Keep it simple.

★

THE RULE OF 5

What following the
Rule of 5 looks like:

BREAKFAST

Scrambled eggs
in coconut oil with
spinach, onion, and
hemp seeds

Sauerkraut

LUNCH

Massaged kale salad with lemon,
avocado and olive oil served with
fermented beetroot

Roasted sweet potato with a little
100% natural almond butter

DINNER

Pan-seared salmon
or chicken

A roasted vegetable finished with
tons of fresh herbs

Leafy lettuce salad with cucumbers
and olives

SNACKS

Can simply be an apple
or carrots, some soup
or a little leftover
roasted broccoli
with lemon

See how there are only a handful of foods in those meals? Your body will be able to
break them down much more easily, leading to less bloating and, again, more energy
for you. You'll be able to focus on the healthier choices without having to think so
hard. I know this won't be possible at every single meal, so don't stress out about it.
Just aim for most of the time and your belly will be feeling better in no time.

SHED RECIPES

Soup: your belly's favourite food! Warm, comforting and the perfect way to get your veggies in, soup saves me during a busy week, especially when I'm overbooked for tea, lunch and dinner dates. Every time I make a big batch of belly-warming soup, I feel like I've set myself up for having the best week possible. Many of these recipes naturally follow the Rule of 5 and are easily adaptable if you're on an elimination diet – especially since none of them contain gluten or dairy!

Kale, White Bean and Fennel Soup
Country Veggie Soup
Spicy Sweet Potato Soup
Bone Broth
Lemony Lentil Soup
Blended Salad Soup
Creamy Vegetable Soup

KALE, WHITE BEAN AND FENNEL SOUP

There are generally good-for-you soups and then there are the gourmet soups, the soups you eat at a restaurant and go, 'Oh my god, this is the best soup I've ever had!'. Usually those restaurant soups have been layered with flavours for hours, sometimes days, using many different cooking techniques. Needless to say, they're VERY labour intensive. With this veggie soup recipe, I've cracked the code on getting the most delicious flavours possible, marrying good for you with totally gourmet, and with the least amount of hands-on work.

MAKES 3–4 SERVINGS

1 head fennel, chopped

1 large onion, sliced

60–120ml extra-virgin olive oil (60ml for a smaller head of fennel and kale, 120ml for larger veggies)

3 or 4 garlic cloves, sliced

2 × 400g cans cannellini beans, drained and rinsed

2–4 tablespoons fresh thyme leaves

Sea salt and freshly ground black pepper

1 litre chicken or vegetable stock, or bone broth (see page 111)

1 bunch fresh kale, stemmed and roughly chopped

Fresh lemon juice (optional)

Chopped fresh parsley (optional)

1 Add the fennel, onion, oil and garlic to a large soup pot.

2 Place over a medium–low heat and mix the vegetables to coat with oil. Cook for 10 minutes, stirring periodically.

3 Add the beans and thyme and season with salt and pepper.

4 Pour in the broth and increase the heat to high.

5 Once the soup is boiling, reduce the heat to low and simmer for 15 minutes.

6 Add the kale and up to 250ml water to cover the vegetables, if needed.

7 Simmer 5 minutes more, until kale is tender.

8 Serve bowls of hot soup with a squeeze of fresh lemon and a sprinkle of parsley if desired.

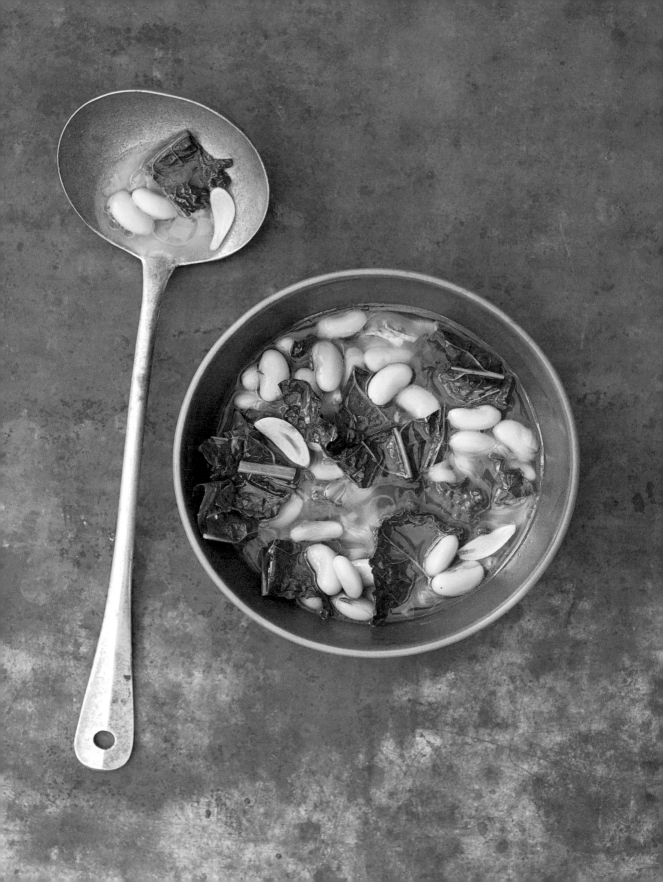

COUNTRY VEGGIE SOUP

This is a classic feel-good soup, packed with flavour from fresh herbs and tons of delicious vegetables. The meaty baby Bella mushrooms and chunky Yukon gold potatoes give this soup a special heartiness that warms you from the inside out. The best part? This soup improves over time, so make a big pot on a Sunday and enjoy it all week long.

MAKES 3 TO 4 SERVINGS

1 large onion, sliced

3 or 4 garlic cloves

1 head fennel, chopped

60–120ml extra-virgin olive oil (60ml for smaller veggies, 120ml for larger ones)

150g carrots, chopped

100g celery, chopped

75g baby Bella mushrooms, sliced

1 small–medium Yukon gold potato, chopped

2–4 tablespoons fresh oregano leaves

1 or 2 bay leaves

Sea salt and freshly ground black pepper

1 litre chicken or vegetable stock, or bone broth (see page 111)

2 corn cobs, shucked and kernels cut off

2 plum tomatoes, chopped

Fresh lemon juice (optional)

Chopped fresh parsley (optional)

1 Add the onion, garlic, fennel and oil to a large soup pot over a medium–low heat and mix the vegetables to coat with oil. Cook for 10 minutes, stirring periodically.

3 Add the carrots, celery, mushrooms, potato, oregano and bay leaves. Season with salt and pepper.

4 Cook for 10 minutes more.

5 Pour in the broth and increase the heat to high.

6 Once the soup is boiling, reduce the heat and simmer it for 10 minutes.

7 Add the corn kernels, tomatoes, and up to 250ml water to cover the vegetables, if needed.

8 Simmer 20 minutes more, until the potato is fork tender.

9 Serve bowls of hot soup with a squeeze of fresh lemon and a sprinkle of parsley if desired.

SPICY SWEET POTATO SOUP

Puréed soups are so calming for the belly and so satisfying to eat. I especially love this recipe served with 'a bird on it' a.k.a. fried egg, a sprinkle of freshly chopped parsley, and a drizzle of olive or truffle oil. When it's served this way, I consider dinner done. If you can't cook, start here. Seriously. This recipe has so few ingredients, tastes amazing, and is pretty much impossible to mess up. All my 'non-cooks' love it. Cayenne pepper adds a kick that starts your metabolism. Plus, sweet potatoes reduce sugar cravings and are high in Vitamins C and D, iron and magnesium – the anti-stress and relaxation mineral.

MAKES 3-4 SERVINGS

1 tablespoon coconut oil

1 onion, sliced

2 garlic cloves, sliced

2 large sweet potatoes, cubed

1 litre chicken or vegetable stock, or bone broth (see page 111)

¼ teaspoon cayenne pepper

Sea salt

1 Heat the oil in a large pot over medium heat.

2 Add the onion and garlic and cook for about 5 minutes, until they are softened.

3 Add the sweet potatoes and stock. Season with the cayenne pepper and salt and bring the pot to a boil.

4 Reduce the heat to low, cover and simmer for 15 minutes, until the potatoes are tender.

5 Purée the soup using an immersion blender or regular blender. If using a countertop blender, purée it in small batches, filling the blender just a bit past half full to avoid spilling.

6 Serve immediately or cover and refrigerate.

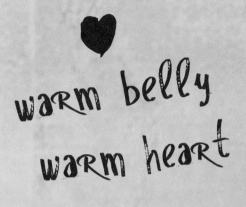

warm belly

warm heart

BONE BROTH

Ahhh, the oh-so-trendy bone broth. Believe it or not, the consumption of bone broth goes way back to our ancestors as a way to get the most out of their precious meat rations. I had learned how to make bone broth in my NYC kitchen over the years but I only perfected it when I visited the magical town of Asheville, NC. The woman teaching us all about bone broth was wearing a loincloth from an animal she hunted, butchered and consumed all by herself. That is definitely the woman you want to learn how to make a proper bone broth from! The key is using tons of bones and cooking them for a long time so all the nutrients leach into the water. This super-powered recipe for a healthy gut has healed many, including myself, from years of unhealthy food (and alcohol!) choices. Try adding turmeric, ginger, garlic or miso when serving for added benefits.

MAKES 6–10 SERVINGS, DEPENDING ON USAGE

1kg chicken bones or 1.8kg chicken parts with meat

4 celery stalks, roughly chopped

4 carrots, roughly chopped

2 onions, quartered

½ bunch fresh dill

1 teaspoon peppercorns

1 teaspoon salt

2 tablespoons unpasteurized apple cider vinegar

7.5cm piece fresh ginger, peeled and roughly chopped

½ fennel bulb, roughly chopped

1 Add all the ingredients to a soup pot or slow cooker, noting that the bones and vegetables should make up the bulk of the pot. Pour in water just to cover them.

2 Cover and bring the pot to a boil or set a slow cooker on high.

3 Reduce the heat to a simmer and continue cooking for at least 3 hours, or overnight in a slow cooker on low. The broth should be dark in colour and rich in flavour when done.

4 Strain the broth and discard the bones and veggies. I'll sometimes push the veggies and herbs against the strainer with the back of a spoon to extract all the broth. Cool and refrigerate it or freeze it for up to 2 months.

NOTE

You can swap the chicken bones for red meat bones, you'll just want to roast those bones first for 25-30 minutes at 190°C/gas mark 5. Fish bones also work great! You can even make a vegetarian version with seaweed using 80g re-hydrated wakame, tons more veggies such as kale and beets and 70g miso paste at the end of cooking.

LEMONY LENTIL SOUP

One of the first recipes I developed for my blog, this is always a hit and fills that perfect 'let's have soup for dinner' slot. I especially love to serve it with a favourite of my husband's and mine, 'Cheesy Bread' – gluten-free bread grilled with butter, sea salt and a hefty serving of nutritional yeast. YUM!

MAKES 3–4 SERVINGS

3 tablespoons extra-virgin olive oil, plus more for drizzling

1 large onion, chopped

2 garlic cloves, very finely chopped

1 tablespoon tomato purée

1 teaspoon ground cumin

½ teaspoon sea salt

¼ teaspoon freshly ground black pepper

Pinch of ground chilli powder or cayenne

1 litre vegetable or chicken stock, or bone broth (see page 111)

200g red lentils

1 large carrot, diced (I usually leave the peel on!)

Juice of 1 lemon

3 tablespoons chopped fresh coriander or parsley, plus extra

1 egg per serving, fried or poached in the soup (optional)

Sprinkle of chopped fresh parsley (optional)

1 In a large pan, heat the oil over a medium–low heat. Add the onion and garlic and sauté until they are golden, about 4–6 minutes.

2 Stir in the tomato purée, cumin, sea salt, pepper and chilli powder or cayenne and sauté for a further 2 minutes.

3 Add the broth, lentils, carrot and 480ml water. Bring to a low boil, then partially cover the pan and turn the heat back to medium–low. Simmer until the lentils are soft, about 30 minutes. Taste and add more sea salt if necessary.

4 Using a handheld or regular blender, purée half the soup then add it back to the pot. The soup can be somewhat chunky or you can purée all of it – up to you!

5 Stir in the lemon juice and chopped herbs.

6 Serve the soup drizzled with extra-virgin olive oil and another sprinkle of fresh herbs.

7 If serving with an egg, crack the eggs into each portion of soup to poach it or add a fried egg on top. Sprinkle with parsley, if using.

BLENDED SALAD SOUP

I got this recipe straight from my mum as she's the queen of gazpacho. In summertime, she makes a vat of it every week, and I feel like it's all I ever see her eat. And why not? Loaded with veggies, easy and light, it's a perfectly refreshing soup that lasts in the fridge all week – and, she says, it gets even better with time.

MAKES 3–4 SERVINGS

1 cucumber, halved, seeded and roughly chopped, but not peeled

2 red peppers, roughly chopped (I typically use 1 red and 1 yellow for colour; any kind but green work – green peppers are unripe and difficult to digest)

4 plum or vine tomatoes, roughly chopped

1 small red onion, roughly chopped

3 garlic cloves, crushed

1.4 litres tomato juice

60ml raw apple cider or balsamic vinegar

60ml extra-virgin olive oil

Sea salt and freshly ground black pepper

Squeeze of lemon juice

1 Put each vegetable separately into a food processor and pulse until it is coarsely chopped. Do not over-process it to a purée! Alternatively, you can chop everything finely with a knife.

2 After each vegetable is processed, combine in a large bowl and add the garlic, tomato juice, vinegar, olive oil and season with sea salt and pepper. Mix well and refrigerate before serving. The longer gazpacho sits, the more the flavours will develop.

3 Squeeze lemon juice on top before serving.

CREAMY VEGETABLE SOUP

I know it's not cool to talk about dieting and weight loss anymore in the happy holistic wellness land, but to be real, this is my secret get-back-on-track soup. Why? Because those 80g of cashews combined with heaps of veggies will fill you up like nobody's business. And because sometimes, even though we may know better, we find ourselves at the end of a pretty long line of not-so-great food choices and want to drop those extra pounds that have crept up on us. So this soup is it. All of the variations work perfectly: I don't even have a favourite!

MAKES 3-4 SERVINGS

80g unsalted cashew nuts

2 tablespoons coconut oil

1 large onion, chopped

2 garlic cloves, chopped

1kg broccoli, cauliflower or tomatoes, chopped

2–3 teaspoons sea salt

½ teaspoon freshly ground black pepper

1 Leave the cashew nuts to soak in a bowl of water for 20 minutes then rinse and drain. (If you don't have 20 minutes, 5 minutes works too!)

2 Warm the oil in a large pan over medium heat.

3 Sauté the onion and garlic until they are tender, about 5 minutes.

4 Add your veggie of choice, enough water to cover, the sea salt and pepper. Simmer for 8–10 minutes, until the vegetables are tender and soft.

5 Transfer the soup to a blender (see Note), working in batches if necessary. Add the cashew nuts and blend until smooth.

6 Taste for seasoning and serve immediately, or let the soup cool then cover and refrigerate.

★
NOTE

If you're not using a Vitamix, wait for the soup to cool before blending. You can use a handheld blender directly in the pan, too.

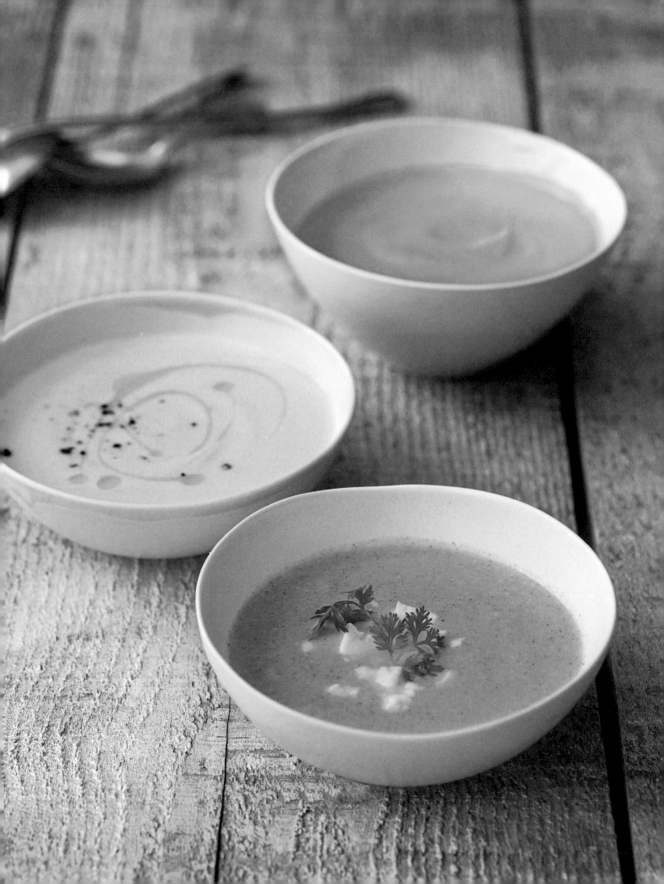

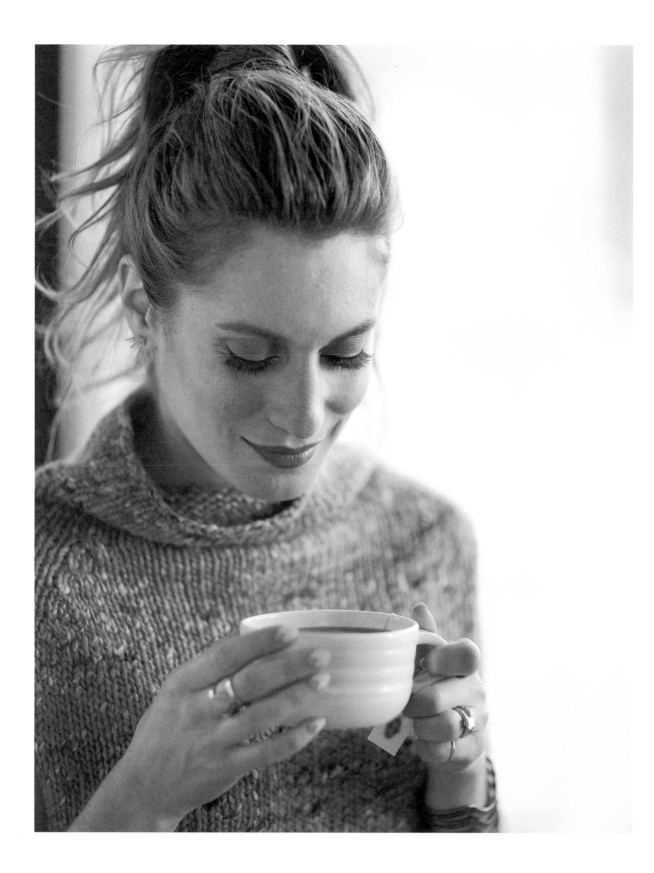

CHAPTER 7

LISTEN

If you've ever spent more than 10 minutes with me, you likely know my love of *Sex and the City*. I know every episode backwards and forwards and pray for the day that there's a game show devoted solely to this particular talent of mine. It was the only box set of DVDs I owned during my years in L.A. and, therefore, the only thing I watched as I self-soothed while eating my second frozen pizza designed to feed a family of four. Anyway, to use a Carrie Bradshaw word, we all have someone in our lives who is a 'frenemy'. They are constantly popping up and you want to hate 'em, but really, deep down, you love them, too.

I like to think of cravings as my favourite frenemy – not quite an enemy, but not really a friend either. Cravings can come to us like needy, aggressive pests, banging at our stomachs just when we don't have time to think straight or the strength to resist. They can make us feel out of control and bullied.

One particular client who comes to mind is Suzanne and her love of old-fashioned, crunchy, salty, sourdough-style pretzels. Suzanne worked for herself as an in-demand and highly paid transcriber. She would spend long days transcribing for her high-level and stressed-out clients. She often had to soothe their fears over deadlines and keep herself calm and focused enough to complete all her work. So what did Suzanne do at the end of her insanely long days of comforting others and pounding away on her laptop? She binged on massive quantities of giant hard pretzels. All that repressed emotion

showed up as cravings and practically spilled out of her with each calming bite.

Clearly she needed another way to approach her cravings. At first we found clarity around her stressful workday and discovered that most of her meals lacked a satisfying crunchy element, such as flaked almonds or raw carrots. We added in some new foods (like naturally salty and nourishing seaweeds), she let go of the overly stressful clients (focusing on the great ones) and upgraded her pretzels to a small serving of sourdough spelt pretzels. And guess what? Suzanne made more money than she ever had before, didn't have to deal with the excessive hours she no longer took on and lost 10 pounds! From frenemy to true ally, her cravings not only helped guide her gut back on track, but also helped her carve a calmer and happier work life.

THE SWEET SIDE OF CRAVINGS

All cravings are really just a kind of communication between your brain and body. And if you know how to listen to them, you can learn how to answer them better. It's my personal belief that cravings are an indicator of something you may actually need that's missing from your diet. Or, they can be a sign of imbalance; a red flag that you are abusing a particular food.

Do you have a crazy amount of cravings? If you feel like your entire life is being controlled by your frenemies, you might be overdoing it

on sugar and sweeteners without realising it. I've noticed that the majority of the women I work with who experience insatiable cravings tend to have an addiction to sweetness and sugar. It happens so easily, for some of us, from infancy. Most foods produced and packaged for children, even if 100 per cent 'natural' from the health food store, are sweetened with at least three different forms of sugar. Sugar is in almost everything – even your barbecued chicken.

Worse yet, these foods are perfectly designed to make you crave them, so you buy more of that particular product. In the mind-blowing Michael Moss article that ran in the *New York Times Magazine* in 2013, 'The Extraordinary Science of Addictive Junk Food', Moss exposed how packaged and processed foods have been scientifically engineered to make us addicted and to trick us into not feeling full. He talked about what food-industry insiders call 'the bliss point'. Basically, it's all about getting you hooked. There are only so many apples you can eat in one sitting, but a whole bag of sweet potato crisps or vegan biscuits? No problem!

Did you know that eating sugar actually makes you crave more sugar? No joke. Eating overly sweet things, especially phony sweet things that contain artificial sweeteners such as sucralose, aspartame (used in diet soda) and even overly processed stevia (a naturally sweet leaf in its original form that is typically mixed with hidden unhealthy sugar substitutes) will trigger your cravings for more sweet. Ever notice that as soon as you finish most packaged 'health' bars, you immediately want another one? Yeah, well, the people that make those bars hope you want another one, too.

The chemicals in artificial sweeteners are digestive nightmares, too. They mess with your gut bacteria and your glucose levels. The microbiome in your belly contains thousands of species and subspecies of gut bacteria that are meant to co-exist and support your digestive function and have a huge impact on your metabolism and immunity. We want a happy and diverse ecosystem of bacteria in there.

Eran Elinav, an immunologist with the Weizmann Institute of Science in Israel and one of the lead researchers in a study written up in the journal *Nature*, spoke about his findings to the mainstream media about what is now being discovered in this massively developing field of study. According to Forbes' rundown of one of the more interesting bits of research, one group of mice was fed a solution

tip

A favourite trick of mine is to add a pinch of sea salt to my sweet recipes instead of sugar. I find this amplifies the flavour and brings everything into balance. Naturally sweet herbs and spices such as mint and cinnamon also do the trick.

CRAVINGS ARE AN OPPORTUNITY TO TUNE INTO OUR BODIES AND HEAR WHAT WE REALLY NEED.

of sugar and another group was given a solution with artificial sweeteners. After 11 weeks, in spite of the fact that the mice in the group with the artificial sweeteners consumed fewer calories, their blood sugar was higher and their weight was the same as the sugar-consuming mice. They used saccharine, aspartame and sucralose separately and each trial yielded the same results.

In order to counter the high blood sugar in the mice taking artificial sweetener (or what I'll call the 'phony sweetener mice'), they had to be given antibiotics. And here is where this stuff gets juicy for a digestive info geek like me: Elinav and his fellow scientists, working on the theory that the fake stuff had screwed with the intestinal bacteria in these mice, performed a faecal transplant, effectively inputting the bacterial ecosystems of the 'phony sweetener mice' into the guts of the mice that had never ingested the phony baloney sugar.

Conclusion? Guess who now had elevated blood sugar? You got it. The mice that had the guts of the 'phony sweetener mice' transplanted into them.

I'm not trying to tell you to go back to that regular soda habit you ditched after you turned 20, but I have a secret I don't usually share: my name is Robyn Youkilis and I am a recovering Diet Coke addict.

When I entered nutrition school as a self-proclaimed healthy individual consuming tuna salad on whole wheat, baked potato chips and buckets of diet iced tea every day, I would patiently wait for my beloved afternoon soda break. I justified it by saying it was only one per day; what harm could it do? My friends were consuming litres of the stuff. At the start of school, I was given the opportunity to work with my own health coach as part of the curriculum. The first order of business during our very first call? Ditch the diet soda habit immediately. It was not up for debate. And so I did. As I chucked that bad habit out of the window (ever notice that some are easy to release just like that while others can take years?), what went most surprisingly with it was my lifelong nighttime grazing behaviour. Those endless rounds from fridge to cabinet to freezer and back again seemed to disappear overnight with this one simple change.

I got off the hamster wheel and haven't had one since.

If the 'good' microbes and bacteria in our guts are imbalanced, our digestive function is impaired, our immune system is impaired and our body's ability to communicate from one part to another is also impaired. That can lead to cravings and hunger at times that don't make sense. This explains why, after my day of consuming so many fake sweeteners and fake foods, I was still trying to feed myself hours into the night. P.S., I also got colds and sinus infections all the time (more proof of my immune system screaming at me).

When our immune system is in distress, we are more likely to get sick or require medications for digestive-related illnesses that stem from this root cause: a jacked-up gut ecosystem that consequently sends our cravings out of whack. As Dr. Martin Blaser explains in his book, *Missing Microbes*, taking antibiotics can strip our stomachs of those healthy bacteria that we need to maintain not just our gut health but also, yes ladies, that other sexy ecosystem of the vagina, a.k.a. your lady parts. Or, as my sister-in-law Whitney charmingly called it as a child, her 'wedgetables'.

Having too much sugar in your diet not only has immediate consequences, including making you constantly think that you need ice cream or, even worse, sugar-free, fat-free frozen yogurt, it also can lead to some stubborn and annoying long-term issues. With time, a sugar addiction can result in candida (an overgrowth of yeast in the vagina) and the yeast infections that go along with it, sleep disorders such as insomnia,

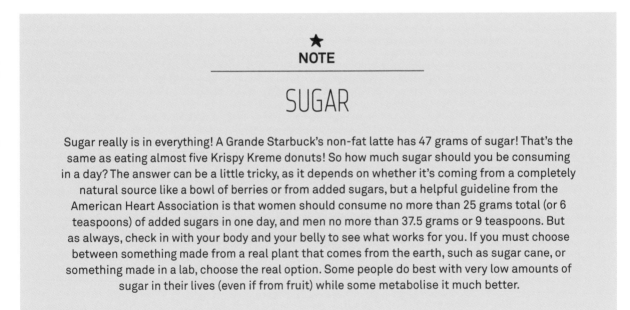

★
NOTE

SUGAR

Sugar really is in everything! A Grande Starbuck's non-fat latte has 47 grams of sugar! That's the same as eating almost five Krispy Kreme donuts! So how much sugar should you be consuming in a day? The answer can be a little tricky, as it depends on whether it's coming from a completely natural source like a bowl of berries or from added sugars, but a helpful guideline from the American Heart Association is that women should consume no more than 25 grams total (or 6 teaspoons) of added sugars in one day, and men no more than 37.5 grams or 9 teaspoons. But as always, check in with your body and your belly to see what works for you. If you must choose between something made from a real plant that comes from the earth, such as sugar cane, or something made in a lab, choose the real option. Some people do best with very low amounts of sugar in their lives (even if from fruit) while some metabolise it much better.

as well as other progressive gut issues. Feeding these types of cravings puts a bandage over what your body is trying to communicate to you, emotionally and physically. We need to do the work to get to the root cause.

Remember when we talked about alkaline balance in the body and pH levels? Excess sugar is also extremely acidic, both in the stomach and in the mouth, where you produce saliva and taste what you're consuming. Over consumption of sugar isn't just giving you cavities, as your dental bill illustrates, it's affecting the ecosystem inside your mouth, where you now know your digestive process begins.

But hey, there is good news here: in slow, gradual change that involves crowding out the less healthy options, choice by choice, and bringing in more of the good, our palate can change. I have a client who, when she began working with me, had an extreme sugar addiction. But as she upgraded the foods she ate on a regular basis and gradually included more and more naturally sweet foods instead of foods loaded with added and processed sugars, things began to taste different to her. She called me in total disbelief with tears of joy after we had been working together for about a year. She had gone to a friend's birthday party and when she tried a dessert that had always been her favourite in the past, her taste buds felt overwhelmed; it was too sweet for her!

WHAT YOUR BODY REALLY NEEDS

A craving can also be a call from your body that it lacks, and needs, a particular nutrient. The problem for us is that the voices that scream 'Eat me! Eat me!' the loudest are usually not giving us what we need and are making us feel like slaves instead. These are the foods that have the most intense flavours: the sweetest, the saltiest, the fattiest.

Cravings can actually be a blessing in disguise, though. Cravings are an opportunity to tune in to our bodies and hear what we really need.

There are four things I ask my clients to check themselves on when it comes to tuning in to intense cravings: water (are you thirsty?), emotions (check in with your feelings, not the fridge), self-sabotage (what happened today with your eating?) and habit (are you just on auto-pilot?).

For example, I used to get tripped up by dessert after dinner. It took a long time for me to realise that dessert was an emotional habit and a memory-based need for me, not a belly-based necessity. One of the ways my brother Paul and I bonded during our teenage years was going to get ice cream together after we had eaten dinner at home. From the time Paul could drive on his own, he took over the activity from our father and it would just be the two of us, going for Vanilla Coke Floats (with extra vanilla syrup, no less).

Once you learn to decode what your body is actually asking for, the cravings will naturally start to dial down and, while they may never completely go away (we always need reminders to tune back in, slow down and check in), they'll be less visceral and intense and perhaps even manageable (code for no big deal).

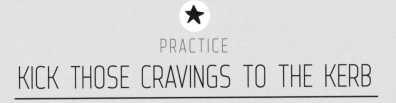

KICK THOSE CRAVINGS TO THE KERB

First, crowd out your less healthy food choices with other upgraded foods and sweet vegetables. This is a helpful philosophy I learnt during my days at the Institute for Integrative Nutrition. Make sure you're eating an abundance of fresh, real and nourishing foods throughout your day, especially naturally sweet vegetables such as sweet potatoes, squashes, onions and beetroot.

Second, experiment with the amount of carbs and protein in your diet. Some of us need more than the usual amount of one or the other.

Third, observe the two-minute rule: when you have a strong craving, set a timer for two minutes and ask yourself what you really want. If you just want something sweet, maybe an apple will do instead of a brownie.

Last, try incorporating a teaspoon of a superfood called spirulina in your diet during the warmer months. Rich in plant-based protein, spirulina is easy to add to smoothies and provides extra protection against cravings.

Keep in mind that our frenemies usually don't just go away overnight. But, as in real life, if you keep saying, 'I can't talk to you today', they will eventually get the hint.

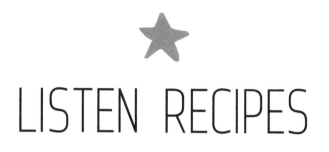

LISTEN RECIPES

Cravings are the body's way of telling us what it needs. These recipes are my healthy upgrades to the most craveable foods: biscuits, pizza, chocolate cake! Yes, you can have a healthier, upgraded chocolate cake, as long as you enjoy every delicious bite.

Coconut Flour Biscuits
Cauliflower Pizza
Carob Yogurt Pudding
Oatmeal-chocolate Chip Powerballs
Coconut Chewies
Pumpkin Muffins
Good Gut Gummies
Chocolate Cake

COCONUT FLOUR BISCUITS

Eager for something 'bready' but confused by all the supposedly healthy bread options out there? Between the long lists of ingredients, multiple kinds of added sugar and difficult-to-digest gluten, traditional shop-bought bread can be a minefield for your digestive system. I would love to bake my own gut-friendly bread but, honestly, I'm not a baker! So, I set out to develop a bread-like recipe that can be whipped up quickly and easily cooked on the hob when a craving hits. I've included varieties to accompany every kind of meal, from breakfast to dessert!

EACH VERSION MAKES 1 OR 2 SERVINGS DEPENDING ON USAGE

BASIC RECIPE

2 eggs

3 tablespoons coconut flour, plus extra
if needed

3 tablespoons coconut oil, melted

Pinch of sea salt

CHEDDAR AND CHIVE

2 tablespoons grated hard goats' cheese

1 tablespoon chopped fresh chives

ITALIAN HERB

1 tablespoon dried Italian seasoning

CHOCOLATE BROWNIE

2 tablespoons maple syrup

2 tablespoons unsweetened cocoa powder

1 Crack the eggs into a bowl and whisk them thoroughly.

2 Add the flour, 2 tablespoons coconut oil and salt, plus the ingredients for your variation of choice, and continue to mix.

3 The batter should be loose, but solid enough to form into small patties. If it's not, add a little more coconut flour.

4 Heat the remaining tablespoon of coconut oil in a frying pan over a medium heat and add your desired amount of the biscuit mix. More mix will yield a bigger 'bun-sized' biscuit while 2 tablespoons will yield a smaller 'snack-style' biscuit.

5 Cook on each side for roughly 2-3 minutes, until they are toasty brown.

6 Serve immediately.

★
NOTE

*Craving buttered toast?
Slice the biscuits in half, add a little butter
and return them to the frying pan on the
sliced side until brown and crisp.*

CAULIFLOWER PIZZA

Cauliflower pizza, let me count the ways that I love thee. Who doesn't crave pizza? Especially when there are pizza joints on almost every block near my home! In my Your Healthiest You community, pizza is everyone's favourite food, so I knew I had to create a version that was better for your belly and your body. With this recipe, you can eat a whole pizza that's made entirely from veggies! Below, I've included a traditional and dairy version; they're both great in their own delicious ways. Traditionally, this recipe has you draining the excess water from the cauliflower in a tea-towel. As you can imagine, that method is quite messy (and really, what are you supposed to do with that tea-towel afterwards with all those cauliflower bits in it?!). I knew that to get my girls in the kitchen, I would need to make the recipe as accessible as possible. My method has you roasting the cauliflower first, which eliminates the tea-towel step and adds an extra-yummy flavour to your pizza pie.

MAKES 2–4 SERVINGS

2 heads cauliflower, chopped into florets

60ml extra-virgin olive oil

2 teaspoons sea salt

1 egg

1 tablespoon ground flax meal

1 teaspoon dried Italian seasoning

4–5 tablespoons nutritional yeast or 750g soft goat's cheese

Toppings of choice

1 Preheat the oven to 200°C/gas mark 6.

2 Place the chopped cauliflower on two baking trays and season it with the oil and sea salt.

3 Roast for 20–25 minutes, until beginning to brown or browned completely (both work fine).

4 Combine the roasted cauliflower in a food processor with the egg and pulse until it is completely ground up. Pulse in the flax meal, Italian seasoning and nutritional yeast or cheese.

5 Line a clean baking tray with greaseproof paper and create two mounds, splitting the dough in half. Mould the dough into a pizza shape (round or square) with your fingers, pressing it down to create a small base roughly 1cm thick. You may need to dip your fingers in a little water to keep them from sticking.

6 Put the pizza bases in the oven and bake for 15 minutes. You can also freeze one of the pizza bases after this step for another pizza night!

7 Flip the base and top it with your favourite toppings. When making a traditional pizza, I'll use tomato sauce, grated hard goats' cheese and some chopped fresh basil. You can also get creative with chutneys, sliced figs, crumbled feta and mint or pesto, any kind of caramelised onions and shredded chicken or prawns.

8 Bake for an additional 15 minutes until the edges are brown and crisp, toppings are heated through and cheese is melted (if using).

9 Cut the pizza into wedges and serve immediately.

CAROB YOGURT PUDDING

I remember having carob chips as a kid when we would go to the local ice cream shop; they were always the alternative chip option and I remember my friends were curious as to why anyone would choose to eat them over regular chips. But I always loved them! Real carob has a delicious, naturally sweet roasted flavour, is free of caffeine and high in Vitamin E and contains gallic acid, which serves as an antibacterial, antiviral, antioxidant, antiseptic and anti-allergen.

MAKES 1 SERVING

240ml plain goat's or sheep's milk yogurt

1 tablespoon carob powder

Pinch of sea salt

¼–½ teaspoon ground cinnamon

Mix the carob powder, salt and cinnamon into the yogurt, spoon into a cup or a bowl and eat!

OATMEAL-CHOCOLATE CHIP POWERBALLS

Would you enjoy a sweet and slightly salty bite that will energise your afternoon and calm those cookie cravings? My dear friend Quinn and I developed this recipe for our blog and show, {Healthy} Cooking Camp. Rather than spiking your blood-sugar levels with traditional biscuits or sweets, these powerballs satisfy a sweet tooth and provide real energy thanks to the oats, nuts and seeds.

MAKES ABOUT 10-12 BALLS

85g rolled oats

115g almond butter

1 tablespoon maple syrup

2 tablespoons dark chocolate chips

1 tablespoon pumpkin seeds

1 tablespoon hemp seeds

½ teaspoon ground cinnamon

¼ teaspoon sea salt

1 Stir together the oats and almond butter in a medium bowl. Stir in the maple syrup, chocolate chips, seeds, cinnamon and salt.

2 Mix until thoroughly combined (you can go ahead and use your hands!). Add some more oats if the mixture feels too wet.

3 Taste the 'batter' and add any additional salt, cinnamon or maple syrup if needed. Spoon out 1-tablespoon portions and shape them into balls. You might need to firmly squeeze them so they keep their shape.

4 Put them in the fridge to set for 30 minutes. Once they're set, cover and keep refrigerated.

COCONUT CHEWIES
CHOCOLATE CHIP, MINT, CINNAMON SPICE, RASPBERRY LEMON

A cross between a biscuit and a macaroon, these are always a party favourite. Coconut is full of nutrients and healthy fats your body uses to power up. The healthy fat will help keep you full and satisfied for much longer than a traditional macaroon or biscuit. Sometimes I'll even whip up all four flavours and make a tray!

MAKES 10–14 CHEWIES

BASE RECIPE

2 egg whites

50g coconut sugar

2 teaspoons vanilla extract

Pinch of sea salt

75g unsweetened desiccated coconut

CHOCOLATE CHIP

45g dark chocolate chips (at least 70% cocoa solids)

MINT

2–4 drops peppermint oil

45g dark chocolate chips (at least 70% cocoa solids, optional if you want a mint chocolate chip version!)

CINNAMON SPICE

1 teaspoon ground cinnamon

1 tablespoon ground flax meal

¼ teaspoon ground ginger

Pinch of cayenne pepper

LEMON RASPBERRY

60g frozen raspberries, defrosted

zest and juice of 1 lemon

1 Preheat the oven to 160°C/gas mark 3.

2 Whisk the egg whites until totally frothy in a large bowl.

3 Add the coconut sugar, vanilla and sea salt. Mix well.

4 Fold in the desiccated coconut and any other ingredients if making different versions.

5 Drop tablespoon-sized balls on a baking sheet lined with parchment paper. Keep the chewies round; do not flatten them.

6 Bake for 20 minutes, until you see a hint of brown on the tops. Allow them to cool completely before diving in. Serve immediately or store in the refrigerator.

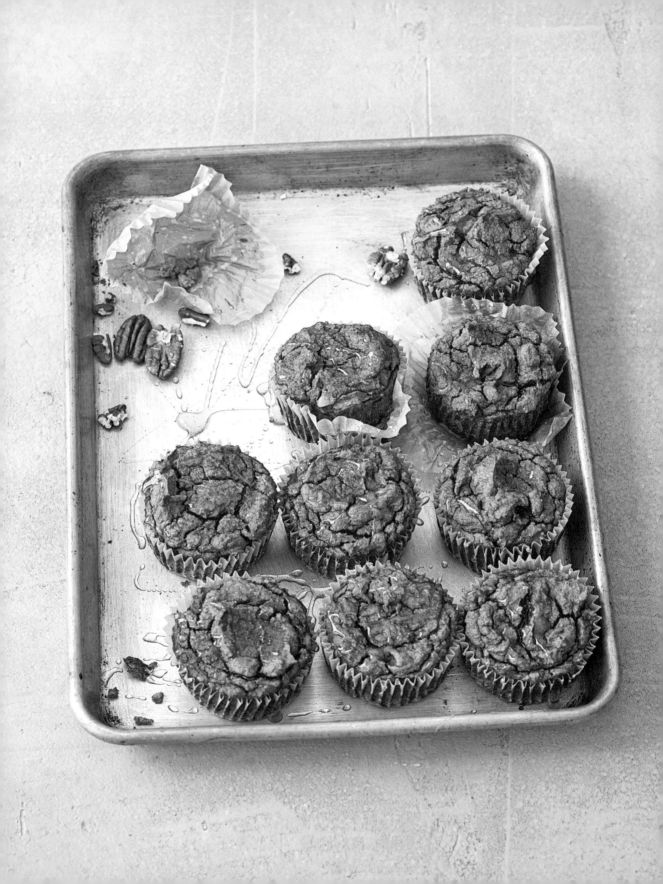

PUMPKIN MUFFINS

Sometimes, you just want a muffin. I remember, when I was growing up on Long Island, I would beg my mum to take me to the neighbourhood deli so I could get a 'fat-free' muffin the size of my head. What? They were 'healthy'! Suuure. Well, I now know better (and you do too!) so I created this truly healthy recipe for any kind of muffin or cupcake craving. I suggest making a big batch of them, storing them in the freezer and then thawing as needed. Just take them out the night before you plan on eating them. If you have the time, cut your muffin in half, butter it up and toast it in a frying pan. I've also served them for dessert with the Coconut Icing from the Chocolate Cake on page 134 and a shaving of real dark chocolate or a sprinkle of cinnamon. Added bonus: kids love them!

MAKES 12 SERVINGS

2 bananas

400g puréed pumpkin

4 eggs

115g unsalted almond butter

55g butter, melted

55g coconut flour

2 teaspoons ground cinnamon

1 teaspoon bicarbonate of soda

1 teaspoon baking powder

2 teaspoons vanilla extract

1 teaspoon sea salt

1 tablespoon ground chia or ground flax seeds (optional)

85g dark chocolate chips or chopped nuts (optional)

1 Preheat the oven to 180°C/gas mark 4. Line a muffin tray with paper cupcake liners.

2 Combine the bananas, puréed pumpkin, eggs, almond butter and butter in a blender, food processor or mixing bowl and mix well, mashing the bananas completely.

3 Add in the coconut flour, cinnamon, bicarbonate of soda, baking powder, vanilla, sea salt, ground chia or flax and chocolate chips or nuts, if using. Mix well.

4 Pour the batter evenly among the cupcake liners.

5 Bake for 30–35 minutes, or until the tops are golden brown.

6 Remove from the oven and allow the muffins to cool.

NOTE

Feel free to serve these with chopped toasted pecans or walnuts and a little drizzle of honey. They're delicious this way!

VARIATION:
BANANA CHOCOLATE-CHIP MUFFINS
Use four bananas, omit the pumpkin purée and include the optional chocolate chips. Bake as directed.

GOOD GUT GUMMIES

I don't know why, but there's something I just LOVE about gummies (jelly sweets). But have you ever looked at the ingredients on the back of a box of fruit snacks or jelly sweets?! Gross! That's why I whipped up these 'good gut' gummies. Gelatin is great for healing your gut as it helps to restore a healthy mucosal lining in the stomach and reduce the amount of inflammation in the body. It's also a pure source of protein, boosts metabolism and reduces heartburn and acid reflux.

SERVINGS DEPENDS ON SIZE AND SHAPE CUT

100g frozen blueberries or raspberries (or a mix of the two)

175ml fresh lemon or lime juice (or a mix of the two)

2–3 teaspoons honey (generally 2 for adults, 3 for kids)

40g unflavoured gelatin

1 Add the berries to a small saucepan over medium heat.

2 Stir the berries and allow them to cook until the liquid is steaming and the berries are plump, about 6–10 minutes.

3 Place the lemon or lime juice, honey and berries into a high-speed blender or food processor and blend until smooth. Remove the lid and allow the mixture to cool slightly.

4 Add the gelatin to the blender and blend again until smooth.

5 Pour the mixture into sweet moulds, or a 23 × 23cm baking tray, and refrigerate for 30 minutes–1 hour.

6 Once the jelly sweets have set, remove them from the moulds or slice them into desired shapes . Store in the refrigerator.

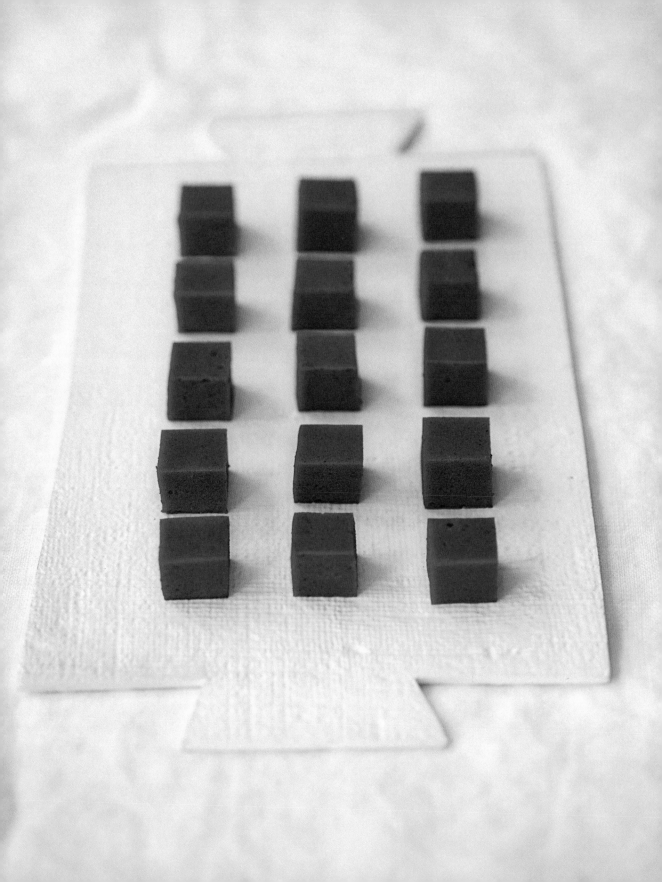

CHOCOLATE CAKE

This book didn't originally have a chocolate cake in it, but when I attended a birthday party and tried this recipe, created by my cooking assistant Gaby, I knew I needed to include it in the book! Our version of a classic chocolate cake, this one contains all good-for-you ingredients without any gluten, refined sugars or flours and nothing funky. There are a lot of steps in this recipe (which is why I didn't originally include it!) but it's worth the work for a special occasion ... like a Tuesday!

MAKES ONE 15CM CAKE

FOR THE CAKE

120ml melted coconut oil, plus extra for greasing

290g blanched almond flour

30g coconut flour

85g raw cacao powder

100g coconut sugar

2 teaspoons bicarbonate of soda

1 teaspoon sea salt

240ml full-fat coconut milk

3 large eggs, at room temperature

2 teaspoons vanilla extract

2 tablespoons raw honey

FOR THE ICING

225g coconut cream

4 tablespoons maple syrup or coconut sugar

25g cocoa powder

1 teaspoon vanilla extract

Pinch of sea salt

FOR THE GARNISH

Coconut flakes

Mint leaves

Strawberries, sliced

1 To make the cake, preheat the oven to 180°C/gas mark 4.

2 Grease the bottom and sides of a 15cm springform cake tin with coconut oil.

3 In a large bowl, mix together the almond flour, coconut flour, raw cacao powder, coconut sugar, bicarbonate of soda and sea salt.

4 In a separate bowl, whisk together the coconut oil, coconut milk, eggs, vanilla and honey.

5 Gently mix the dry ingredients into the wet ingredients.

6 Pour the batter into the prepared tin and bake until a toothpick inserted into the centre comes out clean, about 55–60 minutes.

7 Let the cake cool completely, then cut it horizontally in half.

8 To make the frosting: whisk the coconut cream and the maple syrup or coconut sugar, cocoa powder, vanilla and salt together until smooth. Refrigerate until you're ready to decorate and serve the cake.

10 Put the bottom layer of cake on a plate. Spread a layer of frosting on it. Top with the other half of the cake, finish frosting and decorate.

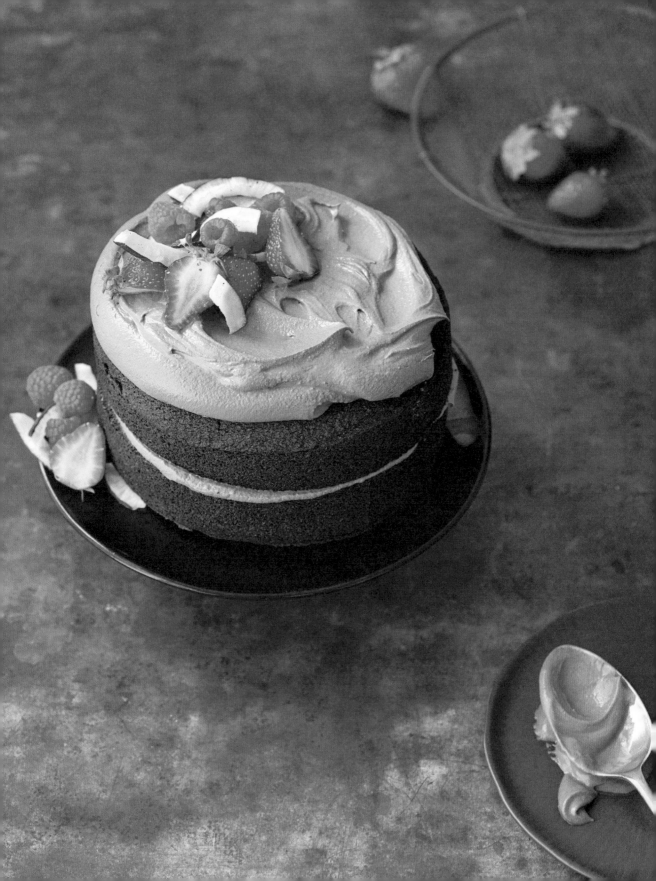

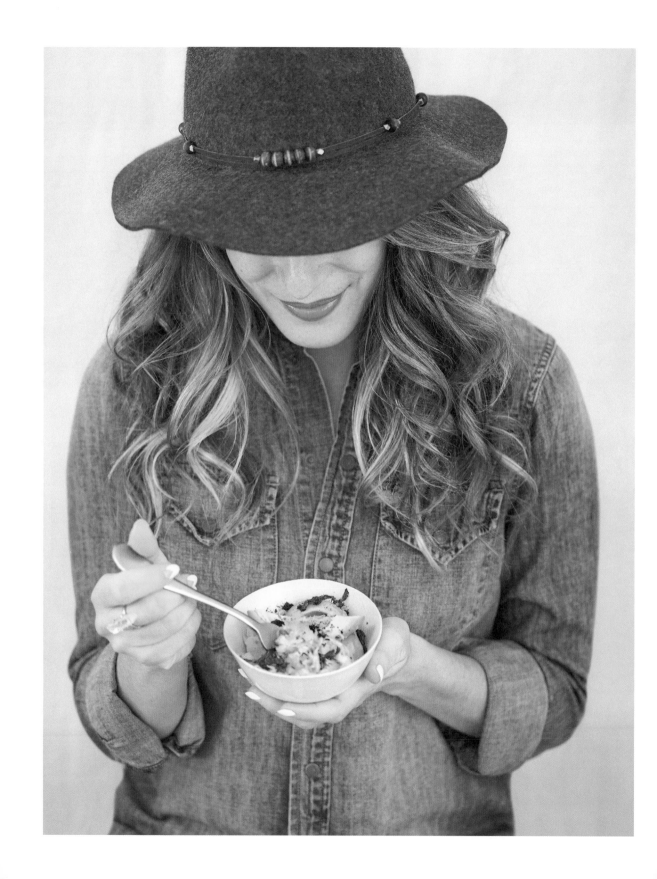

CHAPTER 8

NOURISH

You know by now that eating overly processed foods, those old go-tos that come from a box or bag, is not exactly giving your body what it needs. We know that when our bodies are fed foods that are overly salty or sugary without much realness in there, we wind up feeling hungry all the time. That's because while we have technically been feeding ourselves, our body still signals that it needs more. It needs the actual nutrients and minerals it can use and, until it gets them, you're probably going to feel hungry.

My recipes are all about changing your image of 'roughage' and your desire for the foods that fill you up and satisfy you, from 'Do I have to, Robyn?' to 'Yes, more please!' I believe that you will start to crave the good stuff because it is not just good for you, but also tasty. This is yummy food! I LOVE food and the last thing I want is for you to think about this as an 'I have to if I want to be healthy' obligation. I want you to enjoy eating like I do! I want you to celebrate your appetites, fill your tummies with deliciousness and have fun in your kitchen.

Most of my clients have been in a food rut their entire lives. They focus on familiar go-tos or one particular flavour on the spectrum, such as sweet or salty. If you open the door to let in other tastes (Bitter! Astringent! Sour! Oh my!), you will see that you've been limiting yourself to what you know and shying away from many other foods that you're just not used to.

I grew up eating Peanut Butter Captain Crunch. That is what I associated with deliciousness.

Even though my mum made most of our food from scratch, sugary cereal is still what I wanted and craved. In spite of the fact that I didn't grow up eating from an all-organic, wholefoods kitchen, my taste buds have changed. What's delicious to me now is not exactly what it used to be. I want the same for you. Yes, I still love sweet things, but not the same sweet things as I did, and I treat them as 'sometimes' foods, not what I focus on to carry me through the day.

THE DOWNLOAD ON FERMENTED FOODS

There is a reason fermented foods are on the 'Good Poop List' (page 86). Where greens are a staple of every meal and a portion of every plate, fermented foods are the VIPs at this plate party. Seriously, include them with as many meals a day as possible.

Lacto-fermentation is all about the *Lactobacillus* bacteria, which feeds on sugars to create lactic acid. This bacteria naturally grows on plants as well as in our mouths, lady parts (OK, one lady part in particular) and gastro-intestines. You may recognise 'lacto' and think 'milk' because dairy is one of the many delicious foods where the *Lactobacillus* bacteria exists.

What's so good about lactic acid, you ask? Aside from acting as an agent that preserves food from harmful bacteria, it also protects and even enriches the vitamins and enzyme content of food. When the right kind of bacteria are present in your body, not only are you better able to digest and metabolise the foods that you chew,

but also your body is better able to extract the nutrient content from those foods. More nutrients absorbed from what you're eating = a healthy, more vibrant and more deeply satisfied YOU, in your belly and beyond.

North America is almost the only culture that doesn't regularly include cultured or fermented vegetables in their daily diet. During my many visits to France when my best friend, Lauren, lived in Paris, we became obsessed with the beautiful clay pots of yogurt sold in ordinary grocery stores. Lauren used to save the pots and use them as water cups; they were that pretty. And aside from how charming it was to see yogurt that had been formed in its original tiny pot right next to the six-packs of plastic, sugar-loaded yogurt, eating it was even better. All her life, Lauren had been 'allergic' to dairy. She also believed that she was allergic to fat. Somehow, though, Lauren (probably because of the pretty clay pots) had started to eat this whole-milk, completely natural treat regularly. She found that, first of all, not only did she not gain weight from including some fat in her diet – something she had NEVER done before – but also she was so satisfied after eating one that her appetite was less fierce when it was time for her next meal and … she was not allergic to dairy at all.

tip

If your digestive system doesn't like dairy, there are still plenty of other ways you can meet your calcium needs. Some Go With Your Gut high-calcium foods include sardines, salmon, all dark leafy greens, nuts and seeds.

At least not whole, unpasteurised, unsweetened dairy from a healthily fed and farmed cow.

There is some form of deeply flavourful, culturally distinctive fermented food in every traditional culture on the planet. Sauerkraut, root vegetables and lacto-fermented dairy are commonly consumed in European countries. Asian populations habitually consume pickled vegetables, sauces and kimchi. Soured grains, beer and wine are all fermented foods. Think you've never had a fermented food? If you've partaken in the bread basket at your favourite local restaurant you've had a fermented food. Ditto goes for the wine you had with the meal and the cheese course. Although these are all examples of fermented foods, they're not the ones we're going to focus on for our optimal digestion conversation. If you're transitioning from a diet loaded with excess sugars, the rich sour flavour of fermented foods is going to naturally make you crave less sweet.

So, in a nutshell, the healthy bacteria that grow and colonise in the fermentation process populate your gut when you ingest them. They help your digestion work more efficiently, balance your body – especially if you've ever taken or need to take antibiotics (which literally translates to 'against life') – and are the reason

SO, LADIES, HERE IS MY MANTRA: GET YOUR GREENS ON!

why your gut is so integral to your health: approximately 70–80 per cent of your immune system is inside your digestive system.

You don't need to fully understand this, by the way, to just do it. I want you to make fermented foods for yourself at some point, and in this chapter I show you the simplest ways how. But I get that you're most likely not going to make these fermented foods at home from the start. They are here for you and I do want you to try them, but you can easily buy them, like I do a lot of the time. If you open my fridge, you will see anywhere between five and eight different kinds and colours of fermented veggies. I buy them in the same way I buy new clothes and jewellery for my wardrobe. I think they're fun. And they are the first things I look for whenever I go to a new city, health food shop or farm shop. Every time I make a plate of food, I leave room for them. I Tweet about them, I Instagram them, I talk about them constantly and, most importantly, I eat them! The bottom line is, you need more of these foods in your tummy every single day.

Although my favourite fermentation guru, Sandor Katz (nicknamed Sandorkraut!), travels the world sharing how fermentation creates the most 'compelling flavours' (and as a foodie first, I have to agree), I get that they may not be your first love. One of my favourite little secrets to making fermented veggies craveably great and super mild in flavour for newbies is to mix them with a little fresh lemon juice and mashed avocado. In addition to mellowing the flavour, the fat in the avocado helps to deliver the nutrients into your body. This little trick of a 'recipe' generally makes fermented veggies easy for anyone to consume. If you start with one forkful a meal and work your way up to a 75-gram portion, you will find that once you get used to choosing these foods and tasting them, the easier it will become to choose them more often.

POWERFUL PROBIOTICS

Lacto-fermented foods, contain probiotics from a 100 per cent natural source. Probiotics are live microorganisms that bolster our digestive health. They literally mean 'for life', and we want to include more of them in our diet.

A product may advertise itself as being high in probiotics without actually having the live

cultures you need. What about your fat-free Greek yogurt with packaging that tells you it's 'loaded with probiotics'? It may be, but it's also most likely loaded with excess sugar.

Incidentally, pasteurised and commercially produced yogurt contains only a fraction of the amount of probiotics you need. That yogurt also lacks the important fats that help your body to absorb the nutrient content of certain foods. Fat also helps you feel full and satisfied. Excess sugar, however, creates that good ol' standard – imbalance. Again, you confuse your body. With high-sugar foods, we end up spiking our blood sugar and insulin levels and forcing our bodies to react to a mixed message. Those dramatic spikes can also trigger a fierce appetite, even when you've already eaten.

Probiotic supplements can be a great way to give your body a little backup coverage, but if you take your probiotics in pill form, be aware that not all supplements are created equal. Most mainstream market supplements are heated improperly and are not from a high-quality, trusted source. Also, these pills or capsules usually contain fillers and a fraction of the actual supplements they claim. I am constantly researching and updating my list of recommended probiotics, so be sure to join my newsletter for the most up-to-date information at www.robynyoukilis.com/gutbookbonuses.

I recommend taking probiotic supplements at night. It's when your body is best able to absorb them because your belly and digestive system are most relaxed. Taking a high dose of probiotics at the beginning of your *Go With Your Gut* journey is one of the ways you can eliminate excess yeast and quickly repopulate your gut with friendly bacteria. Not only do probiotics help your belly, they also help your brain. Research shows that depression, anxiety and moodiness have less do with what's going on in your head and more to do with what's going on in your belly.

Since I just took you on a deep dive into fermentation and probiotics, this would be a good time to mention prebiotics too. In a *Huffington Post* article online, the Oxford neurobiologist Dr Philip Burnet put it best. He said, 'Prebiotics are dietary fibres (short chains of sugar molecules) that good bacteria break down and use to multiply. [They] are 'food' for good bacteria already present in the gut. [Consuming] prebiotics therefore increases the numbers of all species of good bacteria (probiotics) in the gut.'

The reason we want to be consuming both pro- and prebiotics is because one feeds the other and, as I've been saying all along, a healthy gut environment is what we're shooting for. Which foods contain prebiotics? You're covered with a comprehensive list in the Prebiotic Foods section of the 'Good Poop List' (page 86). Get ready for dandelion greens, bananas and onions!

Ironically, the primary focus of Dr Burnet's study was the connection between a healthy gut and brain function. Scientists are learning more and more that when our guts are filled with all the good microflora (back to that microbiome

that's such popular science now), our brains work better. And ... this affects our mood! We learned from Dr Burnet's study that people who consumed prebiotics showed less social anxiety than those who did not. How amazing is this information?

THE DOWNLOAD ON GREENS

So, ladies, this one right here is my mantra: Get Your Greens On! Oh, how I love them! Oh how I know you can love them too! I'm talking about every single meal, baby.

Capitalising on variety is really the best way to start loving the good stuff. If you think of greens as just lettuce, you are short-changing yourself and putting an entire world of ingredients into a tiny little box. Buying the same bag of romaine lettuce every week can make anyone bored. There is a virtual green rainbow of options: big, leafy dandelion, Swiss chard, rocket, red leaf lettuce, turnip, broccoli leaf and more. If you are eating a meal and there are no greens involved, you should feel like you are missing the main ingredient. I want you to start to get excited about beautiful, leafy, fresh, earthy greens grown in dirt under the sun. When you get going with my recipes, you'll see how delicious greens can be.

There are many examples of science supporting the fact that the more organic, dark leafy greens we consume, the healthier our bowels and stools are. Greens naturally detoxify your liver, your blood and your respiratory system and are high in calcium, magnesium, iron, potassium, phosphorous, zinc and vitamins A, C, E and K. They also contain tons of fibre and beautiful chlorophyll (making up that lovely green colour). And, people, this food is also filling and 'free!' Meaning, you can eat as much of this as you want! Go nuts! Have fun! You don't have to stress about calories, whether you should or shouldn't eat it; you can go to town! Just be sure to chew thoroughly, of course.

Doesn't it just make sense that your food needs to come from the earth instead of from a cardboard box or a plastic wrapper? I want you to start training your eye in a regular way towards buying greens when you're doing your weekly food shopping.

Let's pause for a sec so you can ask yourself this question: what do you often think about when you're food shopping? What's going on in your head when you're there? What is your current routine and which products you automatically make a beeline for? Can you make a list of your usual go-tos? Are they foods that would fall under the 'Good Poop List' (page 86) or would they be more on the 'Keep it Out of the Home, Office, Car, Everyday Life List' (on page 156)?

Now that you're aware of what you already do, let's set a new foundation. When you walk those aisles, turn off the autopilot for what you're used to buying. Think about this: which variety of the many greens on display looks seasonal and most alive? What's new that you haven't tried? What are you curious about and what are you craving? Greens can be bitter, sweet, savoury and even umami (a savoury taste present in tamari and soy sauce, mushrooms and meat) depending on how you prepare them. The recipes in this book give you options for each of these fabulous tastes.

A kale, spinach, parsley, lemon, cucumber and ginger juice is a hydrating, alkalising, beautifying, super-awesome supplement to any healthy day, but it should not be the primary source of greens in your routine. By all means,

use juices to flood your system with nutrients after a good, sweaty run or as a snack (and it is certainly a happy treat for your digestion). Just consider the following: many juices can be composed of a high percentage of fruit. Basically, if the first ingredient is apples or oranges, you are most likely adding a concentrated amount of sugar into your system and a limited amount of actual greenage.

Also, juices are cooling. They can stimulate the appetite. You may notice that if you choose to juice cleanse and forgo solid foods as an antidote to overconsumption, you wind up bingeing later.

Instead of thinking about eating to lose weight or eating as a reaction to yesterday, go back to those questions we covered in Chapter 1: How do you feel? How hungry are you? What do you need?

We often overlook the temperature of our food except in regards to the weather outside. It's nice to have hot soup on a damp, rainy day, not just because it feels warming. Some studies show that warm foods increase a feeling of fullness, nourishing you from the inside out.

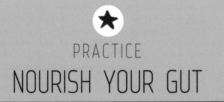

PRACTICE
NOURISH YOUR GUT

Try one new and different leafy green each week and let me know how you like it! Check out the abundance of inspiration and recipe options in the Flow Chapter (see page 88).

Most importantly, try those fermented veggies and get fermenting in your own kitchen! Here are some of my favourite fermenting recipes to get started.

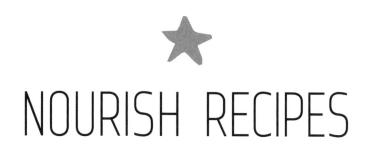

NOURISH RECIPES

Every good *Go With Your Gut* girl needs to try making sauerkraut and fermented beverages at least once or twice in her life! Why make your own fermented foods? Our bodies receive different strains and amounts of beneficial bacteria at different stages of the fermentation process. So if you're always buying your kraut, you likely aren't getting the full range. Plus, they're super fun to make (you feel like a scientist in your own kitchen!) and very cost effective.

Sauerkraut
Go With Your Gut Kraut Snack
Whole Brined Vegetables
Kombucha or Jun
Beetroot Kvass
Shots - Aloe Vera, Immunity Boost,
Better Belly

SAUERKRAUT

Eating raw, fermented sauerkraut is a must for anyone reading this book. If you're unfamiliar with the taste, it's tangy and delicious and can be used in so many different ways. Add it to salads, mix it in stir-fries or eat it straight from the jar! I always include a forkful or two mixed in or on the side of whatever I'm having for lunch or dinner and, of course, with the Superhuman Breakfast.

MAKES ABOUT 600G

1 large head of cabbage, any variety

1 tablespoon sea salt, more if needed

Filtered water, as needed

Additional minor ingredients you can add (make sure your mixture is mostly cabbage):

Thinly sliced apple or pear

Grated beetroot

Onions, thinly sliced

Garlic, finely chopped

OPTIONAL ADD-INS

Caraway seeds

Dried juniper berries

Fresh ginger, peeled and grated

1 Pull off and set aside two outer leaves from the cabbage. Finely shred the remainder.

2 In a large mixing bowl, mix the cabbage with the sea salt by hand. You'll want to spend quite a bit of time on this, until the cabbage starts to get all juicy and you have liquid pooling at the bottom of the bowl. Taste it throughout; it

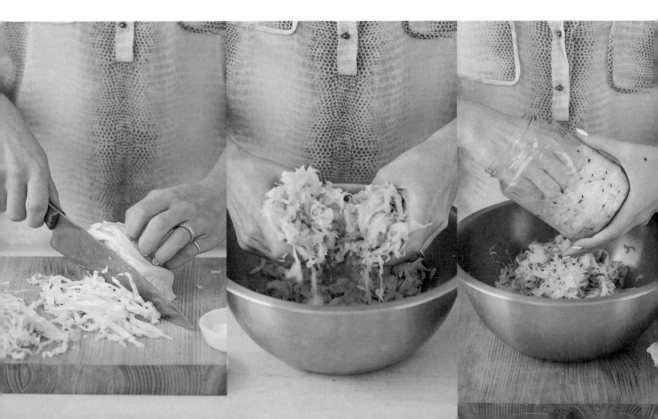

should taste very, very salty. Add any additional ingredients now and mix again.

3 Pack the veggies into a fermenting vessel (a sterilised large class jar with a tight-fitting lid). You'll want to stuff the jar with a few centimetres of cabbage and pack the veggies tightly down, then add another few centimetres and repeat. Liquid should come up and cover the veggies at each stage of the packing and layering. Pack the veggies until you reach the top of the jar, leaving a few centimetres of space. You want to make sure your veggies are below their liquid. If you need to, add a splash of filtered water, or you may need a smaller jar (depending on the size of cabbage used).

4 Layer the top of the veggies with the reserved folded outer cabbage leaves and seal the jar. Leave it at room temperature in a cool, dark place.

5 You'll want to 'burp' your veggies every day or two. Simply unscrew the lid and allow the air to escape. You may want/need to pack your veggies down with your fist again.

6 After about a week, you can taste your kraut. It should taste sour and slightly salty with a tangy flavour and have a nice but strong aroma. If it tastes good, it's good. If it tastes bad, you may need to scrape off the top layer and discard it, then see if the kraut tastes yummy beneath the liquid. Allow it to ferment until your heart desires! I find that anywhere between 10 days and 1 month tastes great (but you can let some ferments go a year or more). Once the taste is to your liking, seal and store it in the fridge for months.

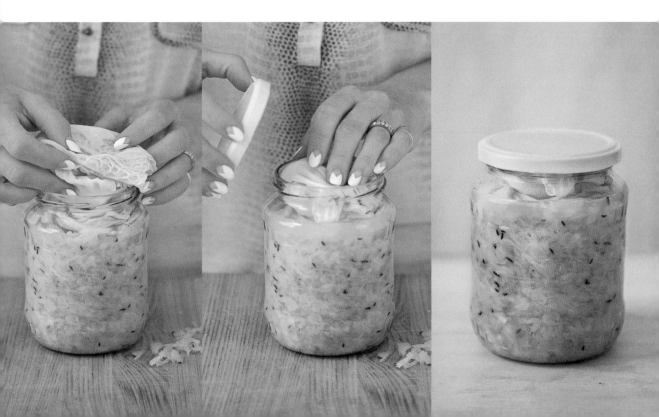

GO WITH YOUR GUT
KRAUT SNACK

Probably my favourite snack, I call this ingredient combo my 'brain bowl'. This was my go-to fuel while working on this book! With brain-fueling healthy fat from the avocado, it kept me clear and energised for hours when I couldn't stop for a full meal. It's perfect as a filling snack or mini meal. This is also a great little dish for kraut newbies; the avocado really mellows its flavour.

MAKES 1 SERVING

40–75g sauerkraut of choice

½ ripe avocado, cubed

Sprinkle of nutritional yeast

Drizzle of olive oil

Sprinkle of gomasio (optional)

Sprinkle of sea salt on avocado, if needed

Layer a plate, bowl or to-go container with your kraut as a base, then add the remaining ingredients on top and eat!

tip

You'll want to use a fresh, clean fork every time you serve your kraut or whole brined vegetables. This keeps the unique bacterias in your mouth from mixing and multiplying in your jar.

WHOLE BRINED VEGETABLES

Delicious, simple and great for your gut, whole brined vegetables are one of the easiest ferments to make. I even got my beloved Aunt Nancy making her own! They're great for snacking on right out of the jar or chopped and added to salads. I also love to mix them into the Mash-Up recipe on page 166.

MAKES 1 LITRE JAR'S WORTH OF VEGETABLES

3 tablespoons sea salt

700ml filtered water

About 400–500g fresh veggies, such as radishes, green beans, beetroots, cauliflower, courgettes, squash, heirloom carrots, lightly washed and de-stemmed

About 2 tablespoons herbs and spices, such as whole peppercorns, lemon zest, dill, mustard seeds, grated fresh ginger

1 Vigorously stir the salt into the water until it dissolves, about 2 minutes depending on the coarseness of the salt.

2 Pack a sterilised 1-litre glass jar (one with a tightly fitting lid) full with the vegetables, herbs and spices.

3 Add the salt water until the veggies are completely submerged, leaving 3–5cm of air at the top. Adjust the level with more or less water as needed.

4 Seal and keep the jar in a cool, dark place for 6–8 days. The time it takes will depend on the taste you want. If you see a lot of 'action' in your jar (lots of bubbles), you'll want to open and close the lid every couple of days.

5 When it reaches the flavour you want, move the jar to the fridge and enjoy! Your veggies will stay good for up to one year.

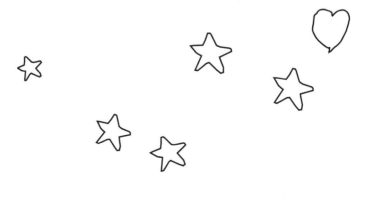

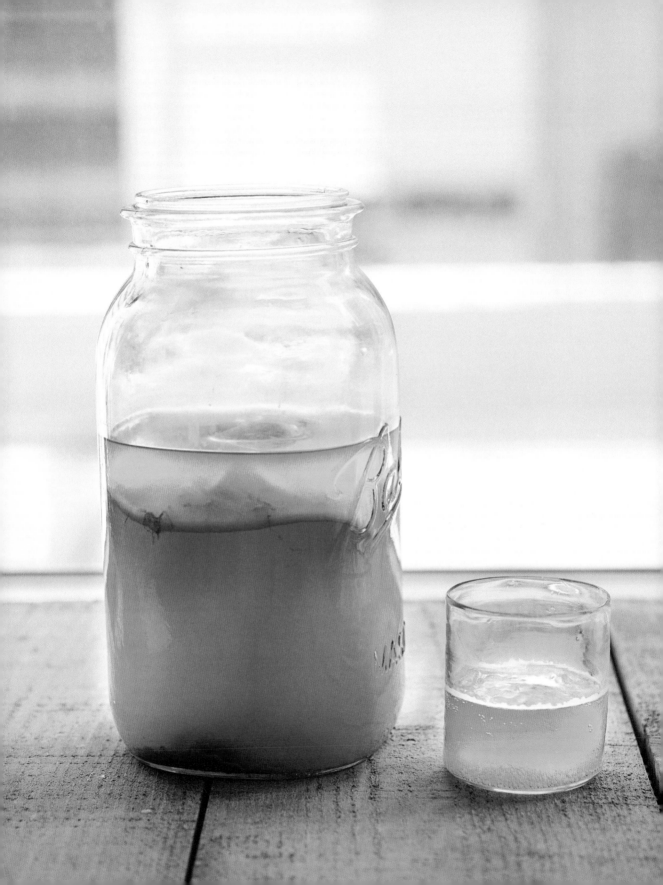

KOMBUCHA OR JUN

Kombucha and jun are popular Asian and Eastern European fermented drinks made with sweet tea and a 'mother' or SCOBY, a symbiotic colony of bacteria and yeast. The 'mother' ferments the tea and creates a delicious and healthy probiotic-filled beverage. Kombucha is a specific type of mother that ferments in black tea and sugar, while jun is a sister SCOBY that has been bred to develop in green tea and honey. You can typically find a mother in your local health food store, or even better, turn to the Go With Your Gut community by signing up for my newsletter at www.robynyoukilis.com/gutbookbonuses to find a friend near you with some SCOBYs to share!

MAKES 1 LITRE

700ml filtered water

50g sugar (for kombucha) or honey (for jun)

1 tablespoon loose black or green tea

or 3 teabags (black for Kombucha, green for Jun)

120ml mature beverage (from your previous batch or wherever you obtained the mother)

Kombucha or jun mother

tip

Storing your SCOBY. If you need to take a break in between batches you can allow the last batch of tea to ferment at room temperature for up to 6 weeks. After 6 weeks, add 50g sugar or honey, cover and place the last batch in the fridge. Every 4–6 weeks you'll need to add more sugar or honey and, ideally, some freshly brewed tea (pour off a little of the last batch) so your SCOBY gets the nourishment it needs.

1 Bring the water and sugar or honey to a boil in a small saucepan.

2 Turn off the heat, add the tea and let it steep for about 15 minutes.

3 Strain the tea into a wide-mouthed vessel (I usually use a jug) and allow the tea to cool.

4 Add the mature beverage and mix.

5 Place the mother on top of the liquid with the opaque side up. Cover it with a dishtowel and allow it to sit in a room temperature spot to ferment. Do not mix the beverage once you add the mother (which likes to be still).

6 Let it ferment for 1–3 weeks. The longer it sits, the more acidic it will become. Taste your beverage and, when it reaches a flavour you like, strain it into jars and place it in the refrigerator.

7 You'll have two mothers left behind: the one you started with and the skin that formed during the fermentation process. You can use the new or old one again and give the other one to a fellow *Go With Your Gut* girl or compost it. Each time you make a new batch, you will have a new mother and the original mother will thicken.

BEETROOT KVASS

Beetroot kvass is a fermented beverage of Ukrainian origin made of beetroot in water with a little bit of salt. I included this healing drink because it's amazing for your digestive system (and especially great for heartburn sufferers) and one of the easiest (and least scary!) ferments to make.

MAKES 1 LITRE

½ bunch of beetroot, any variety, washed, stemmed and roughly chopped

Pinch of sea salt

Filtered water to cover (roughly 700ml)

OPTIONAL ADD-INS

1 tablespoon peeled and grated ginger

¼ cabbage, chopped

¼ onion, chopped

1 Add the beetroot to a sterilised 1-litre glass jar with a tightly fitting lid, leaving about 3–5cm of space at the top of the jar. If using cabbage and onions (these mellow the flavour and make the kvass delicious), use ¼ bunch of beetroot and layer the cabbage and onion in the jar first.

2 Fill the jar with water, leaving a few centimetres of room at the top. Add the salt and seal the jar with a lid.

3 Allow the kvass to ferment at cool room temperature for 3–7 days. It should be a deep red colour and fizzy bubbles should rise to the top. Taste it after 3 days and see if you want a stronger flavour. The rate of fermentation depends on the ingredients used and the temperature. Taste the liquid daily; when it develops a dark colour and tastes right to you (it should be tangy and a bit sour), strain out the beetroot and discard or save and make a second slightly weaker batch of kvass. Drink your fermented kvass daily. I like to enjoy a glass of mine with a squeeze of lemon juice in the afternoon. You can also use this as a base to make beetroot borscht soup or in place of vinegar in any salad dressing.

4 Seal the jar and refrigerate the liquid. Your kvass will stay good for months.

SHOTS

Typically reserved for my high-level coaching clients, these recipes are my best helpful healers. Feeling under the weather? Read below. Not feeling enough flow in your day? I've got a shot for that.

EACH MAKES 1 SERVING

ALOE VERA SHOT

Having digestion troubles? This shot is mainly aloe vera juice, which decreases inflammation in the digestive tract and supports the growth of good bacteria, plus it's guaranteed to help you 'go'. Have one in the morning and one before bed for maximum benefits. I've added the fresh orange juice to mellow the flavour but you can use a little bit of any 100% pure juice.

30–60ml aloe vera juice

½ orange, freshly squeezed

In a glass, mix together the aloe and orange juice and drink! Add a splash of water if you like.

IMMUNITY BOOST

Ahh! My secret winter tonic. This drink is designed to hydrate, soothe and strengthen your gut: the cornerstone of a healthy immune system.

240ml coconut water

2.5cm fresh turmeric root, grated

2.5cm fresh ginger, peeled and grated

Juice of ½ orange

Juice of ½ lemon

1 teaspoon raw local honey

Pinch of cayenne pepper

Freshly ground black pepper

Combine all the ingredients in a blender and mix. Serve and enjoy!

BETTER BELLY SHOT

For those few rare days I go without eating kraut, I'm sure to still sneak in a little probiotic goodness with the juice. This may not be the best-tasting wellness shot (although I love it – it tastes like pickles!), but it'll be over in a sip, I promise!

1 tablespoon sauerkraut juice (from jar)

1–3 tablespoons cold water

Combine the ingredients and shoot!

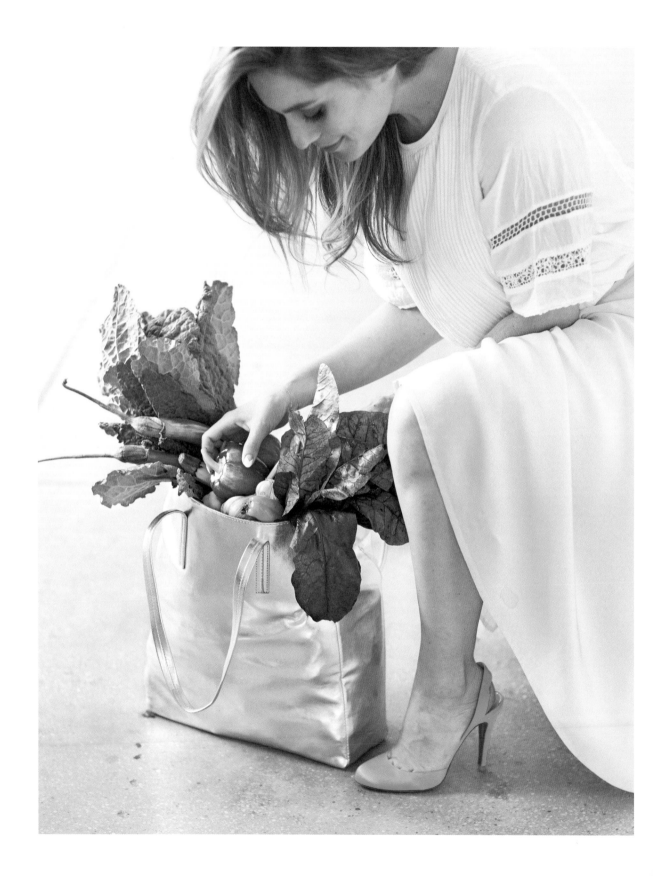

SHOP

So ladies, you are kicking ass now and making kabocha Squash and Kale Tacos (page 50) using organic coconut oil and Himalayan sea salt like a freaking gourmet healthy chef rockstar! You are crowding out the less healthy foods and inviting in more of the optimal. You are breathing throughout your day. You are being mindful and pacing yourself around your plates. You are asking more questions more often and acting on the answers you hear from within. You are chewing your food thoroughly before you swallow. You are restoring the pH balance in your stomach and your mouth. You are healing your gut and repopulating it with friendly bacteria. You are drinking half a litre of water as you shower and get ready for your day in the morning. You are moving your limbs and breaking a sweat even if that means you take 15 minutes to blast some music and bop around in your living room when you have no other time in your day. You are feeling good. Really, really good.

Exit the standard antibiotics and prescription antacids and enter pro/prebiotics and fermented foods at a minimum of two meals per day. Exit the piles of sugar and fake sugar (sorry yeah, we all want to fight this one sometimes) and enter the healthy fats. You are getting your greens on. Now it's time for the really fun part, serious shopping! I'm not talking about a 50 per cent off sale at your favourite online store or outlet centre, I'm talking about your local markets, THE hot spots for my glowing gut gals and all the fresh, seasonal and, most importantly, living produce you will be buying.

MAKING ROOM FOR THE GOOD STUFF

The list of what to stop buying immediately is so easy and obvious you know it already. To take it one step further, my goal is to carve an easier path for these changes to finally happen. I am showing you exactly what to eat, how to shop for, prep and cook alternatives that are so delicious, you will forget you ever craved the things that made you so sick and fed up in the first place.

Here's your **'Keep it Out of the Home, Office, Car, Everyday Life List'**

★ Sugar: this is my KRYPTONITE and likely yours too.

★ Fake sugar: aspartame, saccharine, sucralose, etc.

★ Traditional dairy: milk or milk products from factory-farmed, hormone-injected cows.

Note for dairy: I generally recommend choosing easier-to-digest goats' or sheep's milk-based products over cow's milk.

★ Overly processed foods: beware especially those with a long, unpronounceable name or an incomprehensible ingredient list.

★ Traditionally farmed (meaning not organic!) and produced gluten-containing products: most of us can no longer digest these very well (indeed, as the research piles are building, we wonder whether anyone can!).

★ Poor quality oils:
• Any oil that is partially hydrogenated
• Palm oil
• Rapeseed oil, margarine, soybean oil, vegetable oil

★ Carrageenan: an extract from a red seaweed, it is used as an emulsifier or thickening agent in certain foods we consider to be safe, such as almond milk. Joanne K. Tobacman, M.D., Associate Professor of Clinical Medicine at the University of Illinois at Chicago, has researched this additive and has found that it links to stomach issues, inflammation and 'other malignancies'. It is not a digestible substance.

The 'Good Poop List' from Chapter 5 (page 86) is full of the swaps you will begin to upgrade to and eventually use to replace these items. If these foods don't sound delicious compared to what you have been eating, I defy you to feel that way after making my recipes for one full week. It's more the idea of the foods you think you will miss that bugs you. Once you begin actually tasting and swapping in these new well-seasoned meals, you will want them more and more.

tip

Read your labels! My clients are often surprised by the fact that their favourite 'natural' products contain sugar, artificial ingredients and other not-so-great-for-your-gut stuff, so always read the ingredient label with a careful eye.

GOOD FOOD COSTS MONEY

I know I am asking you to shift your mentality as much as your behaviour regarding food. One of those thought-based transitions that signals a breakdown and breakthrough for so many people in my community is getting over how much healthy food can cost. Fact: good food costs money.

When it comes to food shopping, I officially give you permission to splurge. Whoever told you that food has to be cheap? Whoever said that what you put into your body to fuel and nourish it all day long, every day for the rest of your life should be a disproportionately small allowance compared to everything else in your life? Why would you want to be cheap with your life – with what you can be and do in this world? The question is that big to me.

Chances are, you spend that money already – the money that would make the difference between healthy and unhealthy – in a way that does not lead to your overall well-being, and you know it.

The reality is, it is cheaper to spend money on quality ingredients to cook fresh, simple recipes with just a handful of ingredients than to order a

delivery a few days a week, buy antacids or pay for the inevitable medical prescriptions to treat illnesses that stem from a sick belly.

I've had many clients tell me that hearing about money saved just didn't register for them, because if it's covered by National insurance, it felt like it was free. Part of making this major mental shift is realising that the expense comes out in so many ways you do not even think about – time away from your office or kids to spend a day at the doctor's or even missing out on a party you were so excited about because you are bloated and gassy or constipated.

This is a mindset shift that I believe with all my heart is essential for us to make. I want you to raise your hand and repeat after me: 'I am going to pay what I need to to look and feel my best'. I want you to look for the inherent value in things as opposed to finding the cheapest deal (but we will definitely all cheer with you when the organic berries in your town are on sale!). It's as true of kale as it is of polyester versus cashmere. When it comes to spending, the difference that we are discussing here will wind up being maybe a little bit more, but don't panic; it's OK.

Have you ever played 'let's make a deal' with the cashier at your supermarket? Of course not! But this is actually something you can do at your farmers' market anytime! There was one time I was at the farmers' market when it was closing down and walked away with a ton of free food. The friendly, sweet man who sold me my beautiful bunches of radishes and kale gave me what was left of his turnip greens and a whole bunch of roasting potatoes because he said he didn't want to pack it all up and take it back home. He was smart; he was building a relationship with me. I became a regular customer of his and now go out of my way to buy from him. Incidentally, going back to how much stress affects our bellies, it's way more pleasant and fun to have real interactions when you are picking what will go into your body than it is to search through crazy aisles filled with unhealthy distractions and massive check-out lines. And, of course, it does a gal good to flirt from time to time. Some of those farmers are super cute!

ORGANICS

When it comes to labels like 'organic' or 'organic-like practices', I want you to do your best. Buying organic (or as close as possible) should not be an absolute or an extra layer of pressure, but rather it should be the overall balance of your produce choices, especially those where you consume the outer skin (i.e. berries with thin, fuzzy skin you eat versus a banana with thick skin you discard). Maybe, before, getting fresh seasonal produce at a farmers' market or in the organic section of your usual store felt like a stretch for you. Now, I invite you to see it as part of who you're stepping into being; as something that you do.

I want you to trust that the universe will match you. What I mean by that is, the rest of your daily experiences will also be touched by these choices. Your confidence may rise, your energy and enthusiasm will soar, and how can you measure the impact of that on your job, your interactions and your joy? All of that from one cute little organic apple!

Speaking of apples, though, you will have seen that huge apple in the grocery store that is waxed and shiny and you have seen the ones at the farmers' market that are smaller, dirtier, less round and imperfect. Though the bigger one catches your eye more, its size merely indicates higher water, sugar and carbohydrate

content that will spike your insulin levels and require more effort for your body to digest. That smaller apple was beautifully designed by Mother Nature to have the perfect ratio of skin to inner flesh and the right amount of fibre to help you balance out the sugar. Your body wants those odd-looking, ugly fruits and veggies that are closer to the earth, less manufactured and manhandled and as naturally grown as possible.

Foods that are closer to the earth taste better too – more vibrant and complex. There is real flavour; it's sweeter, juicier and crunchier. Maybe it's just me, but I urge you to do a taste test at home: buy an in-season, organic carrot fashioned with a layer of dirt and top hat of edible greens and a bag of those pre-cut, 'baby' carrots and have your kids, your hubby, or your roommate taste the two together. That farm carrot is sweeter, it has a more nuanced and complex flavour, it's beautiful and it looks like a carrot is supposed to look. And you get a two-for-one vegetable deal when you make pesto out of all those beautiful green leafy tops! Double score!

This is all about getting back to basics on a daily basis: eating naturally produced and farmed food, whole food; eating as many foods as possible in their natural form, from root to stem; cooking simpler meals using simpler preparations and letting the produce shine. If you're going to be cooking with quality oil, salt and pepper, that produce needs to be really good because you actually will taste the vegetables themselves.

FOOD IS ENERGY

OK, you may find this a bit out there, but I totally believe it: there is an energetic property to food. It applies to the act of picking up, selecting and purchasing food that will go into your body. Even further, it follows that if something is harvested and grown with love, at the seasonal time it was supposed to be plucked and picked, it will feel better and agree with us more than something that was grown in darkness or artificial light in mass quantity, sprayed with chemicals and culled by metal machines before it was even ripe.

Plants grow towards sunlight. The sun is a source of energy. You are energy, your belly is energy; you're made of cells and living molecules. The food that goes into your body is converted into your energy. You want that energy clean, light and bright.

Chemicals and pesticides may have made certain foods less expensive and more widely available but they poison our stomachs. Soil used to be so much richer in minerals. The produce we commonly get now is stripped of the valuable micro-organisms that feed the food that feeds us. The good news is that it is getting easier to access local food, from deep suburban to urban environments. A lot of my clients have to drive an hour out of their way to get to their closest wholefood store or farmers' market, but they do it. They even choose to make it an opportunity for a bonding trip with their children. Making your local farmers' market a part of your grocery shopping routine or joining a food co-op or community garden not only connects you to your neighbours in a way that our isolating lifestyles have caused us to forget, but also connects you to a healthy mindset without having to force it.

I belong to a CSA (Community Supported Agriculture) programme where you purchase a farm share at the beginning of the season and are given a local place to pick up your produce each week or, in some cases, it is delivered to

you. In these environments, the seasonal foods are right there in your face; you show up and the right options are waiting for you (see www.communitysupportedagriculture.org.uk).

I love the days I come home from my local CSA with sacks full of seasonal, local veggies and greens and I take the time to lovingly clean and prep them and fill my refrigerator with ready-to-use produce. It's whatever was fresh, abundant and selected for me by the farmer based on the growing season, and I am already well on my way to having a healthy week. It's so much easier to cook for yourself on a regular basis when the ingredients are prepped and waiting for you in your fridge. All you have to do is turn on the oven or hob and get started, even if you drop your knives a few times (like me) or make a giant mess (me again).

I suggest choosing one day a week to take the time to commit to this new healthy and fully sustainable habit. Shop for the week at a place that offers the freshest produce and as soon as you arrive home, wash, chop, dry and refrigerate your beautiful produce to have on hand for the week. Taking the time to chop and otherwise prepare these foods so that they are ready to use will change everything. You won't be too tired to cook; you'll actually be excited.

Being as honest as possible, what are your current food habits? Do you shop for items when you are already hungry? What if you always had what you need to make something fast, easy and super nutritious pre-started at home? Would you start cooking more often? What if you didn't have to think so much? What if it all felt simple and guided for you?

ONE STEP LEADS TO ANOTHER

In our never-ending quest to become our best and healthiest selves, we have become inundated and overburdened with health information. We are thrown all these products, these ideas and rules of what we must or can't do, and told about these food intolerances we may or may not have. What I am laying down for you here in these principles and recipes is a paring down of information. And it holds true whether you're full-time Paleo or 90 per cent raw vegan.

tip

You can clean your produce with this simple wash recipe: 1 tablespoon of apple cider vinegar plus half a litre of water; allow to sit for 5 minutes and then remove the produce and rinse very well.

We ALL need to chew our food completely and that is why mastering that practice is at the centre of everything I teach. I am making this as simple as possible for you. Choose fewer ingredients and care about those ingredients – if there is something you don't want or don't like, skip it for now! I am sharing with you how I eat, how I approach food and how I teach people about food.

We spend a lot of time feeling bad because we are not doing what we know we should be doing for our bodies. You stress over this and, in turn, your digestive system takes the emotional and physical hit. This is why you want to make more choices that result in feeling as good as you can possibly feel. Maybe you don't make these recipes every day. Maybe you still eat a cupcake with sugar icing on occasion. Or maybe you still eat fast food with your kids once a week. But sometimes you choose to make something from this book. Every single time you do that, you feed that part of you that wants to thrive.

When you do what you know is best for you, but is not necessarily what you may want right now, you get infused with the intangible, unshakable knowledge that you are showing up for yourself in the way you know you want to and are meant to. You listen to that instinct that says, 'I want to make a good choice here'. As you listen to that voice, that in turn feeds it and it grows and grows and grows. That's when you start to feel better. That's when your gut can calm down and start thriving. One good choice leads to five great choices. Whatever we put our energy towards grows. The more that those good choices add up, the more your life will add up to the way you want it to look, feel and be. I want you to start seeing everything from the big, whole picture. The more we slow down, connect (and reconnect), stop and ask ourselves what we want, then actually listen to that answer, the better our lives get. It is the same with our digestion. We must pause, place our hands on our bellies and connect. Feel what our bodies tell us, what they want, what they say to us. All it takes is a moment to breathe and take your own pulse. You can feel your internal soothing rhythm reminding you that everything will be OK.

PRACTICE
PANTRY PURGE PARTY!

Out with the old so we can make way for the new! Time to toss and trade up.

Do a thorough pantry and fridge examination. You'll need to throw out all the crap with bad ingredients, i.e. anything that has a super long list, hard-to-pronounce ingredients or has been sitting on your shelf forever. Ditch it or donate it. But just get it out of your home.

Head to the farmers' market or your local health food store and visit my online shop at www.robynyoukilis.com with your new 'Good Poop List' in hand. Focus on adding one or two new foods each time you shop and restocking these better-belly basics from week to week.

SHOP RECIPES

Tired of your same ol' salad or sandwich? Enter the Build-A-Bowl. The humble bowl is a vehicle for tasty, fulfilling and diverse lunches (or dinners). With so many options you will never get bored. Best of all, these recipes come together in a snap once you have your kitchen stocked with all the *Go With Your Gut* staples.

Go With Your Gut Build-a-Bowl
Mashup
Healthy Grains
Let's Get Sprinkling!
Let's Get Dressed!
- Magic Lemon Dressing
- ⟨Healthy⟩ Cooking Camp Special Sauce
- Miso-Turmeric-Tahini Dressing
- Tomato Sauce
- Thai Nut Butter Sauce
- Coriander Yogurt Dressing

GO WITH YOUR GUT
BUILD-A-BOWL

Lunchtime should be one of the easiest and simplest meals for you to assemble, but in a sea of too many options, it can get overwhelming and confusing. To help take the guesswork out of a healthy, easy-to-prepare and filling lunch, I created the Go With Your Gut *Build-a-Bowl. It's totally customisable and totally delicious. Let's get started!*

YOUR BASE – GET YOUR GREENS ON!

I'll be using my 'Good, Better, Best' approach to break this one down. Choose whichever is easiest for you to get started and then add variety as the weeks go on.

GOOD: Boxed pre-washed baby rocket, baby spinach, romaine lettuce or mixed greens. Note: Be sure to buy organic. If you are using spinach, alternate it with other greens often. Spinach is high in oxalic acid, a substance that can deplete calcium from bones in large quantities.

BETTER: Fresh leafy lettuces you cut and store yourself. Chose one to two heads of lettuce each week, depending on how much you personally need (you'll learn this over time). Alternate between red leaf, green leaf, romaine, watercress, lamb's lettuce, rocket, mixed greens and more. When you get home with your greens, immediately chop, wash and dry them (using a salad spinner, if you have one). Store them in a resealable plastic bag with a paper towel or a 'green bag', those special produce bags that extend the life of your fruits and vegetables. Your greens will be ready to go when you are!

BEST: Massaged kale or other dark leafy greens like collards or Swiss chard. Wash and dry the greens. 'Massage' the leaves thoroughly with a little olive oil, salt and lemon juice until they begin to wilt. Use this as the base for the rest of your add-ins. Variation: Rub greens with mashed avocado until thoroughly coated.

VEGGIE ADD-INS – MIX UP THE RAW AND THE COOKED!

You can use any assortment of veggies in the house, from cucumbers to beetroot. I like to use a vegetable peeler for most of my veggies rather than chopping. I find it's more efficient and adds nice variety and texture. I'll sometimes skip the greens base and just start with some steamed veggies and build from there. I love having a warm vegetable component in my bowl.

Suggestions: carrots, cucumbers, peppers, cooked sweet potato or squash, beetroot, sprouts (HIGHLY recommended as they are full of pure, raw energy), raw Jerusalem artichoke, celery, onions, radishes, jicama, celeriac, courgettes, tomatoes, roasted broccoli or cauliflower and any leftover cooked veggies from previous meals.

THE FILLERS

Pick a protein or a grain (if you're eating grains). Try to limit or save grains to one serving in a meal or snack per day. For example, if you're going to a seafood restaurant for dinner, you could choose a wholegrain add-in for your Build-a-Bowl that day.

Protein options: canned tuna, canned, poached or smoked salmon, sardines, white anchovies, any kind of beans (chickpea, cannellini, pinto, haricot, adzuki, mung, etc.), turkey, chicken, tempeh, beef, pork, lamb, eggs, prawns, fish, poultry or meat burgers or Mashup (see page 166).

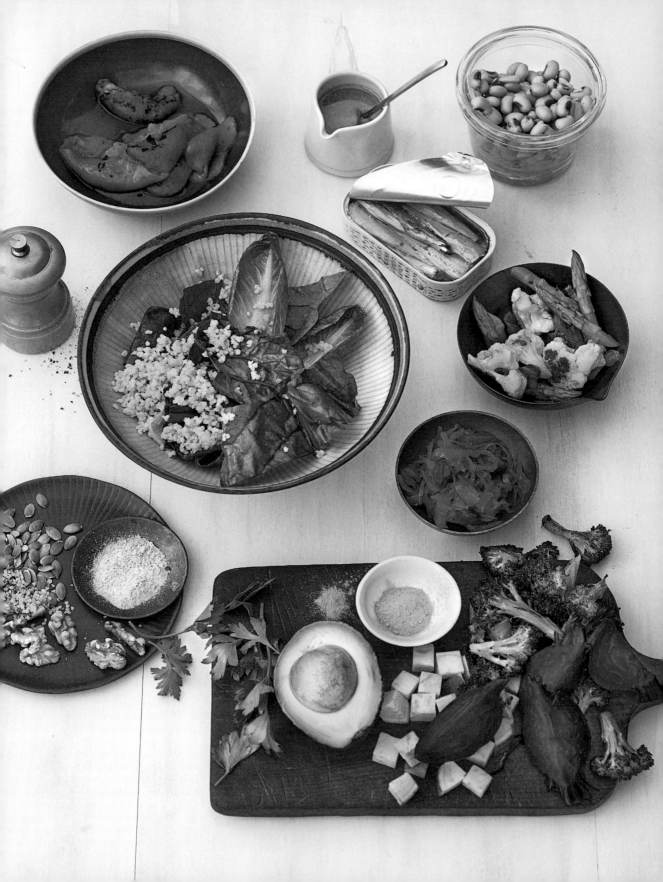

MASHUP
CANNED TUNA, SALMON, MACKEREL, SARDINES, BEANS

This is my go-to recipe for making a meal in less than 5 minutes; I love how this elevates pantry protein staples. This Mashup is delicious on top of a salad, either by itself or with Miso-Turmeric-Tahini dressing (page 169).

MAKES 1 OR 2 SERVINGS

1 can of protein of choice (if using a protein in olive oil, you may not need the olive oil as listed below; if using a protein packed in water, drain water completely and discard)

1–2 tablespoons grated or finely chopped red or white onion, spring onion or shallots

small handful chopped fresh parsley

Zest and juice of ½ lemon or 2 tablespoons apple cider vinegar, red wine vinegar or kraut juice

Sea salt and freshly ground black pepper

40g fermented veggies or chopped whole brined veggies (see page 149)

2 tablespoons Dijon mustard, or more to taste

1–2 tablespoons extra-virgin olive oil (if using a protein packed in water)

ADDITIONAL ADD-IN OPTIONS

1 tablespoon rinsed capers

Chopped roasted peppers

2 tablespoons pitted and chopped olives

1 small cucumber, finely chopped

1 celery stalk, finely chopped

1 Mix everything but the oil in a bowl, leaving your protein as chunky or finely mashed as you like. If you prefer to mellow your raw onions, allow them to soak in the lemon juice or vinegar while you prep the other ingredients, about 3–5 minutes.

2 Add the oil, if using, and mix everything lightly.

3 Cover and refrigerate or enjoy immediately! If I'm low on fresh ingredients, I'll skip the onion, parsley and lemon!

HEALTHY GRAINS

Gluten-free, alkaline for your body and high in protein, these grains (really seeds) contain all nine essential amino acids. I always recommend soaking them whenever possible to make them easier to digest. To soak your grains before cooking, simply leave them covered in water for 20 minutes or up to 8 hours before cooking. Rinse thoroughly and follow the recipe below!

MAKES 4–6 SERVINGS DEPENDING ON USAGE

190g uncooked quinoa or millet

360ml water (for quinoa) or 480ml water (for millet)

2 teaspoons sea salt, more to taste

OPTIONAL ADD-INS

1 or 2 bay leaves

5–10cm kombu, cut into squares

1 Rinse the grain in a fine-mesh sieve until the water runs clear. Drain and transfer it to a medium pan.

2 Add the water and sea salt and bring to a boil. Cover, reduce the heat to medium-low, add any add-ins if using and simmer until the water is absorbed, 15–20 minutes.

3 Remove from the heat and leave to stand for 5 minutes, then uncover and fluff with a fork.

4 Serve immediately or let it cool then cover and refrigerate.

LET'S GET SPRINKLING!

I love boosting the flavour and nutritional value of my bowl by utilising all the easy-to-sprinkle options out there. As these can be stored for long periods of time, I recommend you add a new one to your pantry each time you go to the store. That way you'll have an arsenal of sprinkling options at your fingertips.

HEALTHY FATS: CHOOSE TWO

Seeds (1 tablespoon): be sure to choose raw, such as pumpkin, sunflower, hemp
Nuts (1 tablespoon): raw walnuts or flaked almonds
Add-ins: ¼–½ avocado or 4–6 olives
Dairy (aim for raw): feta or hard or soft goats' cheese

Dairy like: nutritional yeast (an awesome cheesy alternative loaded with B vitamins and my favourite thing on the planet), Daiya cheese

Nutritional boosters (always!): flax meal, chia seeds, dulse or kelp flakes (seaweeds), sliced nori strips, different kinds of raw, fermented veggies (a must!)

Flavour boosters: sea salt, pepper, garlic powder, garlic salt, turmeric, cayenne pepper; fresh herbs such as parsley, basil, oregano and coriander; dried fruits such as raisins, currants, cranberries (make sure they're natural and sulfite free)

LAST STOP – LET'S GET DRESSED!

I recommend one of these three methods for dressing your bowl directly. No need for a recipe, these ingredients can be dumped right into your bowl and mixed together. Full dressing recipe options are given below.

★ Drizzle a mix of olive oil, flax oil, lemon juice and the brine from your fermented veggie jar over your bowl. Season with salt and pepper.

★ A no-oil option: mash avocado with Meyer lemon juice (a delicious tangy and sweet alternative to standard lemon) and a drop or two of pure liquid stevia.

★ Add one part vinegar or lemon juice to two parts oil and a dollop of Dijon mustard. Mix vigorously until well combined with the ingredients in your bowl.

MAGIC LEMON DRESSING

After a single bite, this is the one that makes people say 'What is this dressing? You must gimmie the recipe immediately!' Yep, it's that magical. The secret? Grated raw garlic. When grated finely with a Microplane grater, garlic adds a memorable 'pow' of flavour and is a germ-killing, disease-fighting powerhouse.

MAKES 2–3 SERVINGS

Juice of 1 lemon

2 tablespoons Dijon mustard

1 garlic clove, very finely chopped or grated

4–5 tablespoons extra-virgin olive oil

Sea salt and freshly ground pepper

½ teaspoon maple syrup or honey (optional)

1 Combine the lemon juice, Dijon mustard and garlic in a small bowl.

2 Slowly whisk in the oil until creamy.

3 Season with sea salt and pepper and add maple syrup or honey, if using.

4 Use immediately, or cover and refrigerate.

{HEALTHY} COOKING CAMP SPECIAL SAUCE

Is there anyone in your life who does NOT like to eat their veggies? This is the 'Special Sauce' that will change that completely. Created in the {Healthy} Cooking Camp kitchen, this special sauce is the perfect blend of savoury and sweet. It could go on anything. My favourite way to serve it is over a quinoa salad (which will finally convert any quinoa haters out there!) or on plain steamed leafy greens. I recommend doubling the recipe and using it as a dressing or marinade throughout the week.

MAKES 4–5 SERVINGS DEPENDING ON USAGE

60ml extra-virgin olive oil

60ml apple cider vinegar

60ml maple syrup

120ml low-sodium tamari or coconut aminos

1–2 garlic cloves, very finely chopped or grated

1 Combine all the ingredients in a bowl and whisk together or put them in a jar and shake to mix.

2 Store it refrigerated – maybe in a leftover sauerkraut jar!

MISO-TURMERIC-TAHINI DRESSING

Wanna know a secret? Most of the time, I make really 'boring' dinners. I'll steam some greens, throw some quinoa in the rice cooker, pull out the jar of sauerkraut and open a can of sardines. If I get 'fancy' and have time to get to a fish market, maybe I'll sear a piece of salmon. If I ate that all together on a plate it would be delicious, but, honestly, it might not feel like a 'meal'. So, how do I elevate any meal, add richness and flavour and turn it from 'boring' into truly 'something'? With this Miso-Turmeric-Tahini dressing! Rich and creamy, it brings any plate of food together and adds good-quality fats, from the sesame seeds in the tahini, to your dish.

MAKES 3–4 SERVINGS DEPENDING ON USAGE

1 garlic clove, very finely chopped

1 teaspoon ground turmeric or about 2.5cm turmeric root, grated

1 tablespoon miso paste (optional)

60ml fresh lemon juice

3 tablespoons well-stirred tahini

1–2 tablespoons extra-virgin olive oil

Sea salt and chilli flakes

1 Combine all the ingredients in a bowl and whisk together or blend in a food processor.

2 Add water as needed to thin it to the consistency desired. It will thicken as it sits so I tend to add a little extra water.

3 Use immediately, or cover and refrigerate.

TOMATO SAUCE

Tomato sauce has always been and will always be one of my favourite foods. I guess it's usually referred to as a sauce and not really a 'food' on its own, but I could eat it all by itself! I'll typically serve this over a pile of steamed veggies as my pasta cravings are really tomato sauce cravings. Try it with steamed courgette noodles or kale and grated hard goats' cheese or a hefty sprinkle of nutritional yeast.

MAKES 3–4 SERVINGS DEPENDING ON USAGE

60ml extra-virgin olive oil

2 small onions, chopped

75g carrot, finely chopped

50g celery, finely chopped

2 or 3 garlic cloves, very finely chopped

900g tomatoes, chopped

2 tablespoons tomato purée

½ teaspoon sea salt, plus more to taste

2 tablespoons fresh basil, shredded

1 Heat the oil and onions over medium heat in a large frying pan. Sauté the onions until soft.

2 Add the carrot, celery and garlic and cook for a further 5 minutes.

3 Add the tomatoes, tomato purée and salt and mix well. Continue cooking for 5 minutes.

4 Add 120ml of water and cook for an additional 5 minutes, until all the vegetables are very soft.

5 Garnish with fresh basil. Serve immediately or cool and refrigerate, covered.

THAI NUT BUTTER SAUCE

I was 26, living in L.A. and loving every minute I got to spend with the Dutch rock 'n' roll band that lived below me. They were talented, they loved to have a good time and, most surprisingly, they were incredible cooks. Homemade chips, burritos and many more mind-expanding displays of culinary wizardry made me come knocking. This insanely good Thai peanut dressing was my fave. It was so good, I usually ended up in the kitchen attempting to drink it out of the pot! I've since healthified that recipe and whip it up whenever I'm craving something nutty and rich.

MAKES 1 OR 2 SERVINGS DEPENDING ON USAGE

2 teaspoons grated fresh ginger

2 garlic cloves, very finely chopped or grated

45g peanut, almond or sunflower seed butter

2 tablespoons tamari or coconut aminos

Juice of 1 lime

¼ teaspoon sea salt

1 Combine the ingredients in a bowl and whisk together.

2 Add water until it reaches the desired consistency (usually 2 tablespoons per recipe).

3 Serve immediately, or cover and refrigerate.

CORIANDER YOGURT DRESSING

So you're eating less dairy and your belly is feeling better. Or at least you've switched from cow's milk products to goat's or sheep's milk. Still, I've been there – you honestly just miss cheese and those rich creamy dishes! I get it! Cheese is probably one of my favourite foods on the planet, and I have always been the girl to order extra sour cream. So if you can do dairy without an upset tummy or any of those annoying side-effects including breakouts, this is the perfect sauce for you. This is so versatile it works on anything from Mexican-inspired dishes in place of sour cream to a pasta topping or as a dip for those delicious, savoury Chia Cakes (page 29) or Burgers (page 56).

MAKES 2–3 SERVINGS DEPENDING ON USAGE

180g goats' or sheep's milk plain yogurt

1 tablespoon fresh lemon juice (roughly ½ lemon)

2 tablespoons chopped fresh coriander

Sea salt and freshly ground black pepper

1 In a small bowl, whisk together the yogurt, lemon juice and coriander; season with sea salt and pepper.

2 Add water and stir until the dressing reaches the consistency you want.

3 Serve immediately or cover and refrigerate.

And that's it! You now have the formula for creating your perfect lunch (or dinner!). Change the ingredients from week to week and you'll never get bored. Plus, think about all the space you've cleared up in your brain now that you no longer have to stress over your lunch!

SAMPLE BUILD-A-BOWL IDEAS

WARM PASTA-LIKE DINNER – base of steamed courgettes, fresh tomato sauce and grated raw goat's cheese

SALMON 'NIÇOISE'-STYLE SALAD – base of rocket, cucumbers, steamed green beans, canned or smoked salmon and olives with Magic Lemon Dressing (page 168) and hemp seeds

ZESTY QUINOA BOWL – base of baby kale, quinoa, sardine Mashup and Turmeric-Miso-Tahini Dressing

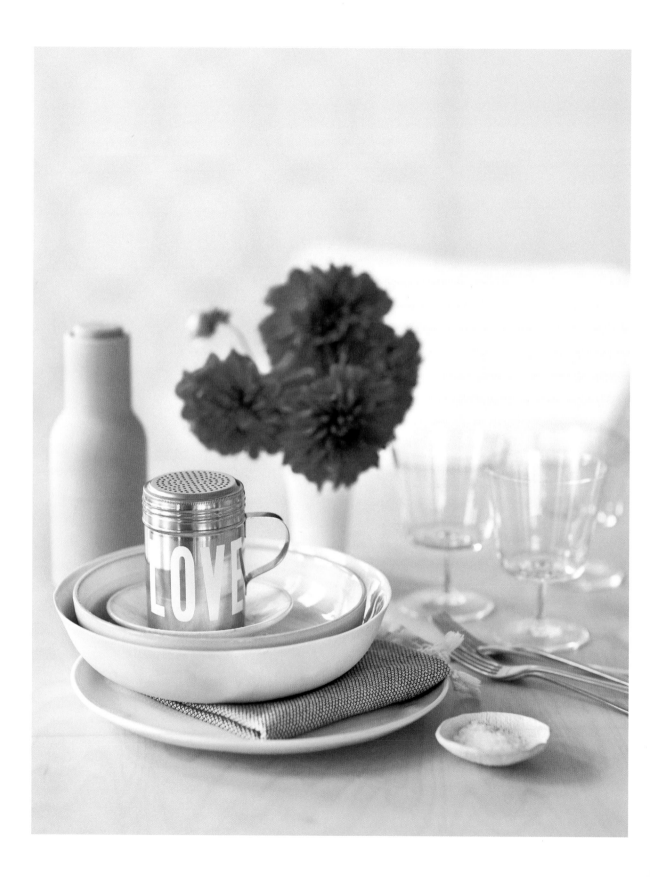

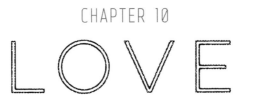

CHAPTER 10

LOVE

What do you love? I don't mean the impressive stuff you put as 'hobbies and interests' on your resumé or online dating profile; I mean the honest-to-goodness things you can't help but turn into a drooling, giggling mess over, like your kids or your family pet, or the TV show you will turn down any super-cool invitation to go and snuggle on your couch and watch – and heaven help anyone who tries to stop you.

Next major question: how do you show yourself love? I bet you have a million different little ways of showing your mother or best friend you love her. What are the habits you have that give love to you?

Is the second question as easy to answer as the first? If you're like most of us, probably not. I want this to be easier for you.

The connection I have been encouraging you to make between your gut (digestive system) and your gut (instinct) is so much stronger when you are used to treating yourself with TLC. But too many of us are so limited in the ways we give that love and the conditions upon which we give it. On the way out of the door to the restaurant, are you pissed at your man if he doesn't tell you that you look nice? My sweet ladies, you can tell yourself! I give you permission to know it and to look in the mirror and say it to your own pretty face! Give yourself a break! What are you waiting for? (By the way, I can't tell you how many nights Scott completely ignores the fabulousness that is a result of numerous outfit changes. And you

know what? I just go ahead and feel like a rock star even if he doesn't get it.)

Newsflash: Loving yourself isn't just about food or being at that magical perfect weight. The more you focus on what you love about yourself and the less judgy you become, the more you will start to look and feel exactly the way you want to.

FOOD EQUALS LOVE

It's so funny the way these things come to us. For me, one of my biggest lessons in learning to love myself came when I fell in love with someone else. I knew I was in love with my husband the first time I cooked for him. To say I went all-out and created a Michelin-star experience is no joke. Something came out of me that I had been pushing off to the side, that my pursuit of a career as an actress and as a hustling documentary film festival producer made me overlook. I am madly, deeply in love with food. I am great at food. I have a talent for inspired, seat-of-the-pants cooking; a natural gift. And that was the first thing that I wanted to share with Scott, to show him. I didn't want him to come and see me stand on a stage and perform. I wanted to make him a meal. I knew if he saw that and loved it, then that meant he 'got' me.

During this time, Scott lived right by the Santa Monica farmers' market in Los Angeles and I was in the first throes of being mad about this guy and would skip down there like a kid in

a candy store and just buy fresh produce like crazy. Before, the way I was cooking for myself looked more like throwing a bag of frozen corn into a pan with fake butter and Parmesan cheese and plating that next to a pre-made, frozen 'veggie' burger. It was just eating food; looking at what I had in the fridge or freezer and making my formula any-kind-of fish (usually from those sad little frozen bags) sautéed with the Old Bay seasoning my mother brought me from her kitchen when I moved to L.A. from New York. But with Scott, I was doing something totally different. Meals like the ultimate spring salad with rocket, fresh broad beans, Meyer lemons, mint and pan-seared scallops. None of it was from a recipe or pre-planned – and it was gorgeous. That is the time when we settled into our routine: I would cook and he would do the dishes while I would hang out, talking to him.

From creating the menus (and obsessing about them all day when I was supposed to be 'working') to buying the ingredients and cooking these crazy weeknight feasts, I realised that this was my language for demonstrating the huge love I felt. And thankfully, Scott came along for the ride.

When I think back, the idea that someone as much in love with food as I am could have a career that did not involve spending 80 per cent of my time cooking and teaching about food is hysterically funny. I mean, I joke all the time that I learned about cooking in the cradle because my mum used to keep my baby bouncer on the kitchen worktop as she cooked. In fact, if you

ever wanted to see the first love of my life, my father, totally blissed out, it was when he was talking about food, sharing a bite of something delicious or bringing our entire family to an amazing restaurant because he had to have us taste that food. I can hear his excited voice practically shouting, 'You have to have a bite of this!' every time I taste something so good that it needs to be shared.

During a trip to L.A. while I was having brunch with my friend, Lesley, I realised that I kept nudging food at her. I must have said a so many times, 'This is so good, please try a bite!' or 'Here, have this'. or 'We should order this! I've heard it's amazing!' As I heard myself doing this, 'Eat this! Eat this! Eat this', I realised again, this was the way my family expressed love. And it is my way of showing love. Feeding someone is my way of saying I am connecting to you from the core of who I really am.

Food is my way of taking care of myself and saying I love you to myself, too. This brought to mind how, when I was growing up, I spent hours in front of the mini TV on our kitchen worktop eating bowl after bowl of Peanut Butter Captain Crunch cereal. In spite of how many times my mother tried to stop me, I pulled my chair so tight up to that screen that there was a permanent dent in the rubbish bin where the chair pressed against it. If my mother called me to do something like clean up my room or do my homework, I was protected because 'I'm eating!'. It was my way of carving out time that was all mine. I was my own boss because I was eating.

THANK YOUR STOMACH.
THANK YOUR BELLY.
LET IT OUT,
LET IT BE A PART OF YOU.

I was in my own space, not having to think or deal, peacefully blissed-out.

LOVE YOURSELF UP

When it comes to the ways we show our love – whether it's to those we care about or to care for ourselves, there are powerful and beautiful ways to do it and there are ways that don't really make us feel the way we want to feel.

We all do this with food. We use it to show love, care and connection, but we also use it to self-soothe and create a bubble of time that belongs to us. Thankfully, once we are able to make this connection, we can learn other more productive ways to care for and soothe ourselves. You can give yourself this relaxation, this release and personal space and time to just chill and ooze into nothing, without using food to do it.

Here are my suggestions for ways to show yourself love, to look out for your mind and body, without using food:

★ Breathing exercise (see page 17)

★ Having a date with yourself

★ Setting up an altar

★ Taking a bath

★ Finding the rituals that are non-food related such as: going for a walk around the block; meeting a friend for a 'fiver' (a quick break) to walk and talk; lying on the floor and feeling the comfort and support beneath you; learning a new hobby for your hands, such as knitting or drawing; or swapping your favourite club seat for a rocking chair. (Note that it's impossible to eat while rocking AND it reminds you of being a little one. Really what is more soothing than literally rocking yourself?)

It's strange that we withhold love from ourselves if we don't like our weight. Your stomach does so much hard work for you. It takes everything you give it and even when you give it harmful foods, it does its very best to use and handle them. We have talked about what happens when your body has to do extra work because you give it unchewed or toxic food. Why blame your body?

How about this instead:
Thank your stomach. Thank your belly. Let it out, let it be a part of you. Place your hand on it as you thank it. Love it so it can love you back.

I don't want to sound totally hippie dippy (or maybe I do), but I don't think it's too 'out there' to

say that everything carries an energy. You can feel if your partner is off or even if your boss doesn't say anything; you can tell by the vibe you're getting or the expression on their face if they are angry with you. Your body is the same way. Your body feels, responds and connects to what you say to it.

Creating beautiful food for Scott and myself was my way into self-care and self-love, in part because that process was about me learning to celebrate one of my strengths, my cooking. I want you to find your own way in. Maybe you have a visual eye and you decide to get yourself beautiful plates with a pattern that makes you smile when you look at them. Maybe you will start plating your weeknight meals for one in a way that looks elegant to you. Light a candle.

Put on some music. Give yourself some time with what you created. Put the leftovers away when you've served yourself. Practise the 123 Food Freedom Tool (see page 19). Sit down and say thanks. Or, maybe you start by plating your take-aways. Take care to set your space at your table no matter what you're eating. Serve your tea in a beautiful cup or mug.

Love is not just reserved for when you win an award or fit into a size down. Love is not just for other people or expensive shoes. Don't hold it back from yourself. Your body will respond when you start killing it with kindness.

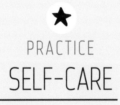

PRACTICE

SELF-CARE

Make a list of 20 self-care practices that you can turn to at night or at weekends. These can include a bath, going for a walk around the block, a hot towel scrub, closing your eyes and deeply breathing for 1 minute and so on. (One note: Make sure the things on this list are actually things you really want to do, not just what you think you should be doing.)

Bring some love into your kitchen. Is your kitchen a place where you want to be? Do you have any personal items in there that make you smile when you see them? A client of mine completely transformed her cooking experience when she hung two beautifully framed enlarged photos – one of her cooking in the kitchen with her mama as a little girl and the other dining at the table with her family's typical weeknight spread. She hung an adorable apron with the cutest pattern. Making this space so filled with things that made her feel so good, made her want to spend time there. Showing herself love through making meals with real, whole foods soon became her favourite thing to do.

LOVE RECIPES

One of the easiest ways to love yourself is to take time each day to slow down and enjoy the present moment. My favourite way to pause is by making tea. The process of stepping aside from whatever craziness you have going on to make yourself a warm cup is so healing and soothing. Not only will your belly thank you for nourishing it with these gut-healing beverages, but you will also feel more connected to yourself by taking this break.

Everyday Soother

Sugar Craving Calmer

Get'er Going Drink

Super Powers Tea

After-Dinner Drink

EVERYDAY SOOTHER

If your digestion feel a bit sluggish, or you overindulged the night before, this gut tonic will help clean out your system and get everything moving. Make sure your water is super hot to get maximum clean-out benefits.

MAKES 1 SERVING

Small handful of fresh mint leaves, torn

1 teaspoon freshly grated ginger

Juice of ½ lemon (optional)

1 Bring 240ml water to a boil in a small saucepan. Add the mint leaves and turn off the heat.

2 Squeeze the juice from the grated ginger into a mug. Remove the mint leaves from the water, discard and pour the boiling water in your mug over the ginger juice. Stir in the lemon juice, if using.

3 Enjoy.

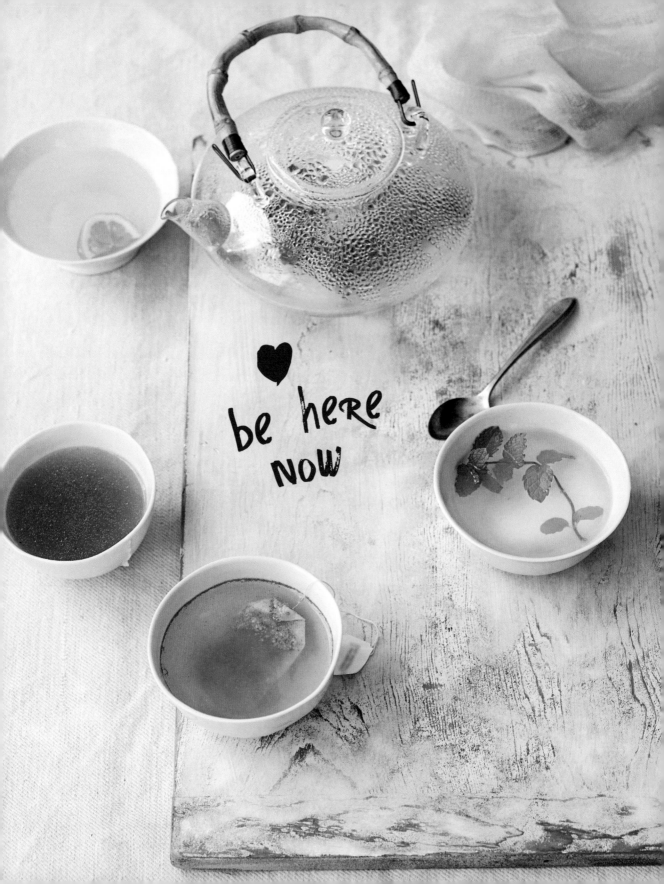

SUGAR CRAVING CALMER

Sweet cravings out of control? This soothing drink will help you feel like you've had a delicious treat and help balance your blood sugar levels.

MAKES 1 SERVING

480ml boiling water

1 bag ginger tea

Juice of ½ lemon

1 teaspoon ground cinnamon, or more to taste

1 Stir together all the ingredients and let the tea steep for 5 minutes.

2 Remove the tea bag and enjoy! Aim to have 2–3 cups per day.

GET 'ER GOING DRINK

OK, this may seem insanely simple to be included in this book as a 'recipe', but drinking hot water with lemon daily will change your life. Try it for 1 week and let me know how your morning flow is going.

MAKES 1 SERVING

Juice of 1 lemon

1 cup hot water

Add lemon juice to hot water and drink.

SUPER POWERS TEA

Stuck in a coffee rut? Try this super powers tea. It's energising, anti-inflammatory and gets your metabolism (and brain!) going. I usually make a pot of it first thing in the morning – after my hot lemon water, of course!

MAKES 1 OR 2 SERVINGS

1–2 teaspoons loose yerba mate tea

¼ teaspoon ground turmeric

Pinch of ground cayenne pepper

Grind of freshly ground black pepper

Ground cinnamon – as much as you like

½ teaspoon maca powder (optional)

1 teaspoon coconut oil

1 Bring about 500ml water to a boil in a saucepan (enough to fill your loose-leaf tea pot).

2 Combine all the tea ingredients in a tea-steeping basket.

3 Add the boiling water. Allow the tea to steep for 2–5 minutes.

4 Pour and drink!

AFTER-DINNER DRINK

A perfect post-meal digestive aid, this tea helps alleviate bloating and gas and calms tummy ache.

MAKES 1 SERVING

240ml boiling water

½ teaspoon fennel seeds

2 teaspoons dried mint leaf or 1 mint tea bag

Pinch of ground ginger or ½ teaspoon freshly grated ginger (optional)

1 teaspoon grass-fed gelatin powder (optional)

1 Add all the ingredients except the gelatin to a large mug. Cover and allow to steep for 5 minutes.

2 Remove the cover, strain if desired and stir in the gelatin powder if using. Sip and enjoy.

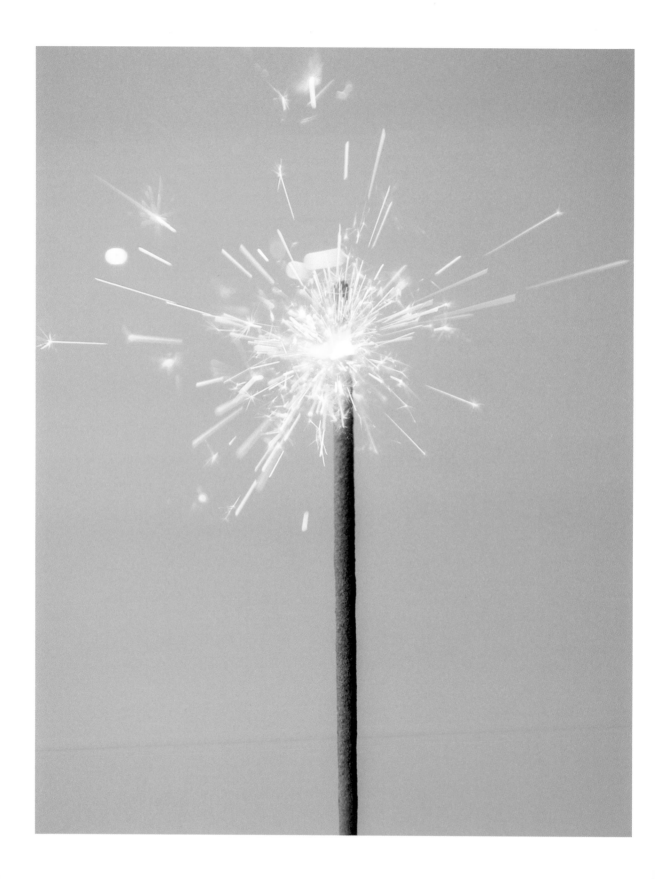

CHAPTER 11

SPARKLE

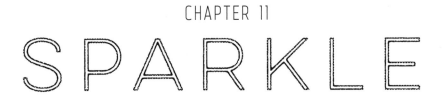

Guess what? You are responsible for the solution to what ails you. I am not here to sell you the idea that this pretty girl or, for that matter, any particular book or guru, diet protocol or drastic cleanse holds the answer. My whole mission is to empower you to be the best possible guardian for your own well-being.

You are a smart cookie. You know which foods and behaviours make you feel good. What gave you a bellyache when you were 8 years old may still leave you sitting on the couch next to your significant other doing your best not to toot in a volume that sends them running and screaming from your side. But, over time, our bodies' reactions to different foods change as well.

I was left out of the raw apple experience throughout my childhood. I could not enjoy one without a severe allergic reaction. I longed to taste those different varieties when autumn came and my whole family went apple picking in Vermont, or know what they tasted like without my entire mouth turning into a puckered attack of itchiness. Lo and behold, that allergy disappeared in my late twenties. Whether it was a product of time and the natural cycle of allergies, or totally in line with completely cleaning up my diet, who knows? But, your body knows. And no one knows your body better than you do.

I don't want to sound too cutesie, but when I got into the topic of how to 'go', it was a natural progression in my mind towards what it means to flow. To fix our bellies is to allow flow. Shift the focus away from the external bullshit – our weight, our wrinkles or spots, our hair – that distracts us from what's really important. Focusing on fixing our bellies first enables the rest of our body to function at its most efficient, to go from blocked to beautiful.

When I was a little girl, my mother would often give me an option at the beginning of the day: 'Do you want to do this today, or do you want to do that today?' My answer was always the same: 'I want to do both and here's how.' I would then proceed to lay out a plan for how we could make it all happen with ease and flow.

Somehow, I was connected to this gut intuition that said, 'How can I figure this problem out? How can I allow for the pieces that were meant to fall into place?'

When you make decisions from that place – when your life comes from that basis of knowing 'What do I want? What do I need right now? What's coming up for me? How do I want to feel?' – you create your day, your life, your experience, from a charged foundation.

You have been there. You have experienced those moments when everything falls in line and you feel calm, inspired and guided in your belly. In those moments, you have felt a sense of magic. This is something we have the ability to connect to every single day, and it directly relates to digestion.

It's hard to feel great from a fog, when there is a dirty screen over your life. It is hard to feel those gut hits, that intuition from your core. It is hard to hear, see and know where you are supposed to be, where you are supposed to go, what you are supposed to be doing. Cleaning up your gut allows you to tap into that sense of connection to your innermost self and intuition much more readily. You are in a state of connection.

You can create your day around feeling how you want to feel, being who you want to be and making (but really allowing) what you want to happen, happen. Now, with the community we have built, you have support.

Wasn't there a meeting at work or a date with the man who became your husband or just a small moment when you knew you were absolutely on fire and you knew exactly what to say? When you are in that place of an initial spark, it charges all that surrounds you. What I am all about and what I want you to take away, if nothing else, is this: when you are in a state of connection with your gut, your centre, and when you are consistently listening, checking in and taking time to breathe into your body and life, then you are able to tap into an intuitive power – you are in a state of being that makes these sparkle moments occur all the time.

Take a moment to answer this. I want you to write it out. How do you want to feel? Ask yourself, 'what is blocked in my body? What is blocked in my life? What do I need to shift to

feel more joy? What do I need to let go of?' Here and now comes the great leap. I want you to start from a place of feeling as if you are totally healthy and happy. Decide that who you are now, already, is the healthiest ideal of who you want to be – someone who cooks her meal instead of eating it out of the container, a Salsa dancer, a doubles tennis player, someone who doesn't stress about fitting into a dress...

How would you run your day and how would you choose for yourself if you already were EXACTLY as you wanted to be?

Your weight is often a physical manifestation of your behaviours and what you eat. Changing how you experience your food (chewing, breathing, being with your plate), cleaning up your food, cooking more, adding in more well-belly foods, connecting with your true self and holding that vision means that as you begin to feel better, your weight will naturally align with the body you are meant to have. This truly happens from the inside out, from your guts to your growth as a human being. Your physical weight may not actually change, but your body will begin to feel so unbelievably different to you.

Most important of all is that you remember that you are a living, breathing being connected to the world, to the galaxy. The ocean, plants, trees and sun need to be fed and need to absorb energy in order to give it. We are the same.

After years of experimenting on myself, hundreds of client success stories, paying attention to what feels good, what tastes good, what works and doesn't, I've discovered the habits that make me feel my best. I feel better able to connect to this energy and to my food. When you begin to use your own common sense, backed up by knowledge you learn from sources you trust, and by tuning into your own gut instinct instead of trusting a label that tells you something is 'healthy', you have begun to make the most powerful connection.

The digestive system runs on a cycle just like Mother Nature does. There are certain times of year when grounding foods (such as beetroot, onions, sweet potatoes and squashes) make us feel right and others when lighter, airy foods (spicy rocket, watercress, fennel, daikon radishes) are what we really need. The more in touch we are with those instincts, the less we will be driven by cravings for the highly processed foods that are formulated to act like drugs.

We need to understand that there is no willpower. There is only one healthy choice, from our guts, that leads to the next healthy choice. Each step we take puts us back in the driver's seat. And there is where we have all the power. Real transformation is not about 'never again'. It is about making these connections more often. Intuition, to me, is not something we have to buy or acquire. It is the most natural, accessible source we have, that wave of knowing that comes from your belly.

Connecting to your intuitive voice and hearing it more clearly can come from simply getting quiet. It could be as easy as putting your hand on your heart and taking a full breath into your belly...

Slowing down ...

Taking a second ...

Taking a breath and checking in.

The path of cleaning up what you put into your belly is a path to connecting to your gut intuition. You cannot separate one from the other. And when you are in that place of connection, those are the moments you feel most alive. When you are guided by that inner resource, that purest place of you, your whole life expands.

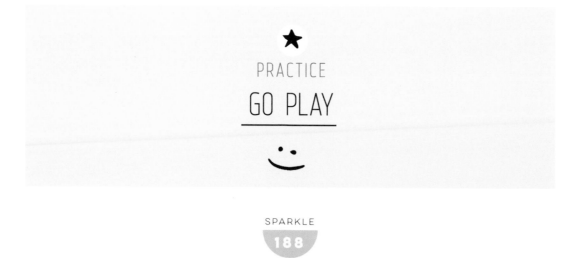

★

PRACTICE
GO PLAY

:)

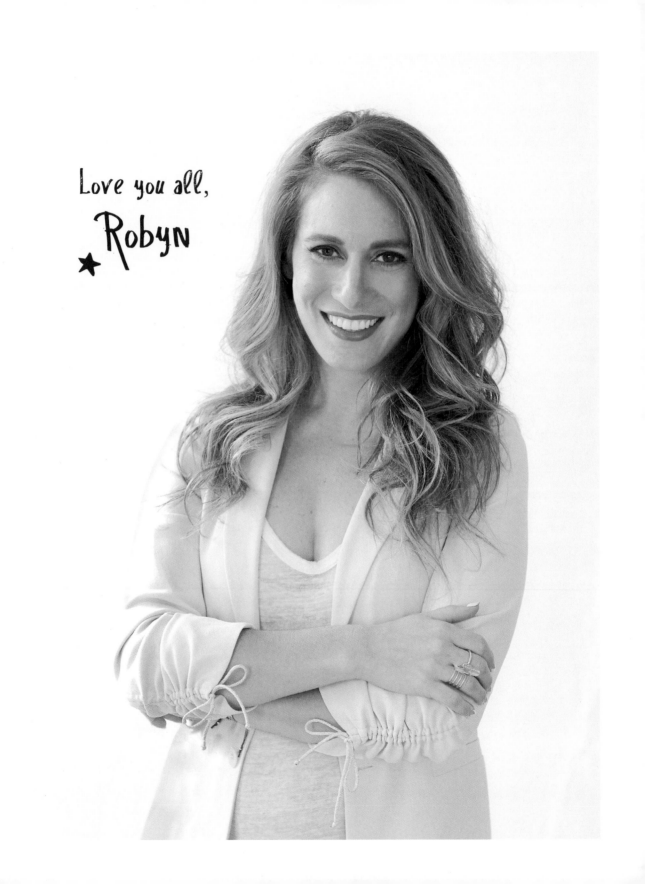

Love you all,

★ Robyn

INDEX

ACKNOWLEDGEMENTS

How can you possibly thank everyone? I'll try to get through this and not cry into my sauerkraut.

Thank you to my parents Marion and Mel for seeing the star in me and for letting me follow my intuition (even when it was less than convenient). Thank you dad for our shared love of food and soft pretzels. I hope you are enjoying all the bagels and schmaltz in the world beyond this one. And mom, thanks for making me try everything (I didn't have to like it, I just had to try it) and always letting me mix the bowl. I could not love you more; you mean everything to me.

And for my coming of age partner-in-crime, my brother, Paul. Thanks for teaching me that it was totally normal to have gourmet lunches when the other kids were merely eating sandwiches and for always pushing me to be a better person in this world. I love you, Jess and little Mel. May he one day enjoy something besides four foods and Benihana.

And for the rest of my family – you all taught me that food is nothing without connection and family and I love you all so much. Aunt Nancy, Uncle Bruce, Andi and Daniel. Aunt Linda, Andrea, Aunt Lanie, Julie, Paul and Marcie. Love to my sisters Lori (thanks for fielding four million cooking q's from LA!), Patty, Penny and all the girlies.

To the other side of my family, the one I was lucky enough to marry into. Thank you for loving me and the mediocre homemade challah I brought the first time I met you. Thank you for supporting me, laughing with me and at me. Claudia, Bob, Whitney, Andrew, Terry and Michaela, you make me feel like I won the family lottery. Because I did.

My friends, especially all my Syracuse girls, Cat, Jess and Jamie and the rest of the Phi's. Thank you Loni, Sophie, Tricia, Lesley, Jess Scheer, Catter, Buncher, Dave, Donna, Laurent and everyone in Scott's Cornell and home crews, I love you all.

My Institute for Integrative Nutrition family and founder Joshua Rosenthal. To my IIN girls Marisa and Elisabeth for believing in me from the moment we met and making me feel like I can do anything. Thank you to all my wellness colleagues and mentors. Gabby Bernstein, for the brilliant forword and for being such an incredible and supportive friend and inspiration. Laura Hames Franklin for teaching me that magic is real. Quinn Asteak for being the Pep to my Salt and for spending a million hours in the kitchen and on-camera with me.

Thank you to my 'sister' and chief collaborator Lauren Seligman for all your committed hard work and editorial help. This book would not be what it is without you and your sheer brilliance. You are a beauty in person and a genius on the page.

Thank you to the people who literally made this book possible. To everyone at Kyle Books for 'getting' me and my vision. Kyle, you are the coolest person I know. Thank you Anja Schmidt for bringing me into the Kyle Books family. Thank you Jessica Goodman, my editor. I'm so grateful for your incredible work on this book baby but even more so for your support and encouragement of this first time author. You made the impossible possible and trusted my gut instincts every step of the way.

Thank you to my agents Sarah Passick and Celeste Fine (who shaped this book before I could even see it). Thank you to my manager Mark Turner and to Ron Longe. Thank you Gaby Kassin, who made the recipes in this beast of a book doable and fun. Thank you to my book team, you elevated this project beyond my wildest dreams, especially my insanely talented and ever-elegant photographer, Ellen Silverman, Nora Singley, Alistair Turnbull and their styling teams and Nicky Collings for your beautiful design. Thank you Amalia Moscoso and Leila Wolford. You are true artists. Thank you to my brilliant lawyer Mikey Glazer for going above and beyond at every opportunity.

Thank you to my team past and present, Emily Kristofferson, Tiffany Manley, Li Panetta and Emily Nachazel. Thank you to every single one of my clients, for believing in me and for our work together, for your transformations inside and out and for every brilliant a-ha moment we've ever shared. You are all the stars in my sky.

And finally my husband, Scott, the best gut instinct of my lifetime. You are the reason I can be who I am today. That I can take risks. That I can explore the world. That I can love so deeply it makes my shoulders shake and my heart quiver. Thank you for always saying you love whatever I cook (except that one time when a balsamic glaze went very, very wrong) and for supporting this book through every tear, frustrating moment and glorious success. I know it's been a long ride and I know it wasn't easy. You are my heart and joy in this crazy world. I love you.